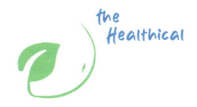

the Healthical

Reduce

A GUIDE TO PREVENT CHILDHOOD OBESITY

Author
Sunanda Rathi

Co-Author
Aashish S Rathi

Copyright © 2023

Dr. Sunanda Rathi
Aashish S Rathi

All rights reserved. No part of this publication may be reproduced, distributed, or transmitted in any form or by any means, including photocopying, recording, or any electronic or mechanical methods, without the prior permission of the author, in case of brief quotations embodied in critical reviews and certain other non-commercial uses permitted by copyright law.

Yoga Protocol given under Integrated Approach of Yoga Therapy is designed and validated by author Dr Rathi. It is her research study that the copyright holder reserves all rights, or holds for its own use. Three Dimensions Yoga Postures have been designed by Chiranjeev Animation Studio as per the requirements of Author Dr Rathi, Animation Pvt. Ltd. holds copyrights for all creatives and diet plan designed especially for this book.

For permission requests, write to the author at the address given below.
ISBN : 978-81-19682-96-6

Any references real people, or real places are used fictitiously. Names, characters and places are products of the author's imagination.

Published by: Beeja House
First Printing Edition 2023
Printed By: Repro Books Limited.
Author Email : yogainitiatives@gmail.com
info@thehealthical.com

www.thehealthical.com

Dedication

To
The Almighty,
Guide, Mentor,
Family Members,
Staff & Students, Friends & Well-wishers.

This book is dedicated to the children of today and the leaders of tomorrow, whose health and happiness are of utmost importance.

To the young minds struggling with the burden of obesity, may this book serve as a guiding light on their journey to wellness through the transformative power of yoga.

This book is dedicated to every child, every parent, every educator, and every guardian on the journey to conquer obesity through yoga and nourishing food habits.

Let us build a world where health, harmony, and happiness flourish for generations to come.

Turn the page to read and follow the sequence to practice, slowly you will find solutions. You will find significant changes within...

Lead Magnet

GET YOUR FREE GIFT! TRATAKA TECHNIQUES

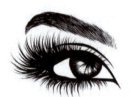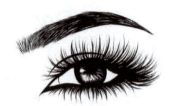

The COVID-19 pandemic has forced schools and universities not only in India but also around the world, to suspend physical classrooms and shift to online classes. Connecting teachers with students through digital platforms and necessary software using laptops or phones is the latest transition in education trying to eradicate the physical need of teachers or classrooms. Virtual classes are going to be part of students' education. This changing trend in education can have a harmful effect on the eyes. Do you agree that there is a need to protect against eye strain?

GET YOUR FREE GIFT! TRATAKA TECHNIQUES

Tratak is a type of yogic sadhana that helps a person to increase concentration, boost confidence, and develop a positive attitude towards life. This can be done by anyone and everyone. It removes bad thoughts and negativity from one's mind and brings out positive vibes.

It's a holistic treatment that nurtures both the physical and mental realms. Regular practice cultivates a sense of inner calm and balance, making it an effective tool for managing anxiety and promoting emotional well-being. By engaging in this practice, children can unlock their inner potential, fostering a profound connection with themselves and the world around them. As the eyes learn to gaze beyond the physical, Tratak unveils the path to a deeper understanding of the self.

TRATAKA KRIYA

"Where the gaze deepens, the mind enlightens."

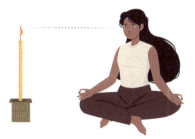

A Sanskrit word, Trataka means "to gaze steadily." Trataka is a practice similar to mindful meditation which comes from ancient yogic visual concentration practices

Benefits of TRATAKA

1. Purifies the eyes and strengthens the eye muscles by exercising them to focus on a point.
2. Corrects short-sightedness.
3. Improves vision, concentration, and memory.
4. Cures sleep-related disorders such as a headache, insomnia.
5. Fixing the gaze the restless mind comes to a halt.

Scan the QR Code to download the google form, fill in the information, and use the "Trataka Technique," you can learn ancient scientific techniques to protect your eyes, which helps purify the eyes and strengthens the eye muscles by exercising them to focus on a point. The session will be online. Time slots will be allotted by the office.

Reduce

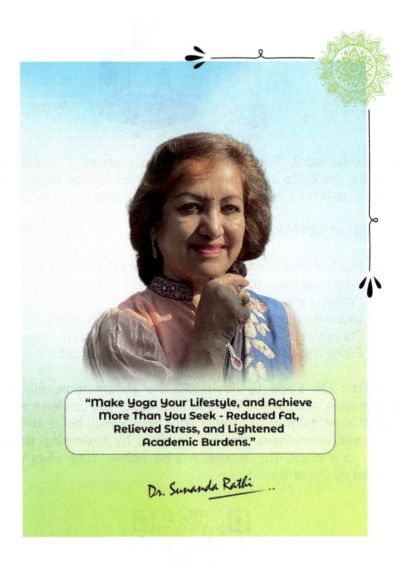

Table of Contents

Author's Desk : Dr. Sunanda Rathi	05
Co-Author's Desk : Aashish S Rathi	07
Forward :	
Acharya Swami Ramdev ji	09
Dr. H.R. Nagendra - Guruji	10
Dr. R. Nagarathna - Didi	11
Mentor Shri. Ramkumar Rathi	12
Testimonial : Dr. Sanjay Malpani	13
Acknowledgment	15

Part A : YOG FOR OBESITY

Chapter 1 : Introduction	17
Chapter 2 : Obesity as per Ancient Indian Literature	21
Chapter 3 : Etiology of Obesity: Causes (Based on Research Study)	23
Chapter 4 : What is Yog & its Benefits in Daily Life	28
Chapter 5 : Integrated Approach of Yog Therapy IAYT	32

Part B : IMPORTANCE OF DIET

Chapter 6 : Healthy and Balanced Diet	123
Chapter 7 : Summary	155
Reference	157
Author's Bio	162

From Authors Desk:
Dr. Sunanda Rathi

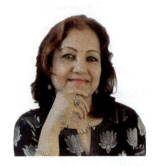

Dear Readers,

It is with great joy and enthusiasm that I present to you my latest creation, "Reduce – A Guide to Prevent Childhood Obesity." As an author and a passionate yoga researcher for health and well-being, this book holds a special place in my heart.

Through extensive research and personal experiences, I have come to realize the critical importance of addressing childhood obesity in our society. The alarming rise in childhood obesity rates is not just a statistic; it represents the potential health and emotional challenges faced by our young generation.

In writing this book, my goal is to offer a comprehensive and practical guide to combat child obesity through the powerful combination of yoga and mindful eating habits. I firmly believe that yoga is not just a physical exercise; it is a holistic approach that nurtures the mind, body, and spirit.

Within these pages, you will find scientifically-backed yoga protocols and an Integrated Approach to Yoga Therapy, IAYT. specifically tailored to address child and adolescent obesity. Moreover, Aashish S Rathi, our co-author has given valuable insights on fostering healthier food habits, empowering parents, educators, and caregivers to lead by example.

It is my sincere hope that " Reduce – A Guide to Prevent Childhood Obesity " serves as a beacon of hope for children, parents, and educators alike. Let us come together to embrace the wisdom of yoga, instil mindful eating habits, and create a healthier world for our children.

Thank you for embarking on this transformative journey with me. Together, let's make a positive impact and empower the younger generation to lead a life filled with health, happiness, and harmony.

With warmest regards,

Sunandas Rathi..

> *"Yoga is the journey of the self, through the self, to the self."*
>
> The Bhagavad Gita

From Co-Authors Desk:
Aashish S Rathi

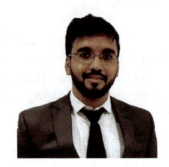

The phrase, "you are what you eat" has been around for quite some time, and for good reason. The food we consume not only affects our physical health but also our mental wellbeing. In other words, what you eat is what you think.

Research has shown that certain foods can impact our brain chemistry, leading to changes in our mood and behavior. Our eating habits can also affect our mindset and perspective on life. Eating a healthy, balanced diet and incorporating Satvik food into our diet can make us feel more energized, motivated, and optimistic.

Satvik food is considered to be a holistic approach to eating, as it promotes overall health and well-being. It is believed to balance the body and mind, and to prevent and heal various diseases. On the other hand, consuming unhealthy food, processed or junk food can lead to feelings of guilt, shame, and negativity. Processed food or junk food is typically high in calories, unhealthy fats, salt, and sugar, and contains artificial additives and preservatives that can cause various health problems, including obesity, diabetes, heart disease, and cancer.

Along with the 60-minute research-based yoga protocol suggested by Dr. Sunanda Rathi, I believe that we as a parent play an important role in shaping our children's overall development because we are an influencer to them. We can help our children develop healthy eating habits that will benefit their health in the long run by creating a positive eating environment and being good role models. Children are keen observers, perceive quickly, and prefer to imitate their parents. Overall, good eating habits can help children develop a strong foundation for a successful and fulfilling future.

In the book I have focused on how to set good eating habits and have a balanced diet that can help the child develop improved health, better academic performance, a strong work ethic, and improved social skills and increased self-confidence.

"*Understanding the vital role of food and diet is equally important. Our habits evolve, change being constant in life. Your adaptability to these changes is key to achieving your goals.*"

Acharya Swami Ramdev Ji

Founder of Patanjali Yogpeeth Haridwar

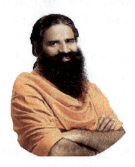

"It brings me immense pleasure & bliss to extend my heartfelt blessings to the creation of the book, "A Guide to Prevent Child Obesity through Scientific Yog Protocol & Diet Habits," authored by Dr. Sunanda Rathi & co-authored by Mr. Aashish S Rathi. This endeavor, penned by visionaries in the field of yog & wellness, holds immense promise in the realm of holistic well-being. Childhood obesity is a pressing concern in our contemporary society, affecting not just physical health but also mental & emotional well-being. Yog protocol & balanced dietary habits, as elucidated in this book, is an effective antidote to this challenge. Meticulous blend of yogic exercises & dietary recommendations, has the potential to steer young minds towards a healthier, more vibrant existence. As I traverse my own journey in spreading the virtues of yogasana & pranayama practices to the masses, I am delighted to witness authors like Dr. Sunanda & Aashish contributing expertise to the well-being of society. The holistic approach outlined in this book resonates deeply with the ethos of yog – a path that transcends physical postures to encompass mental & spiritual harmony. My message is clear: don't just read the book; immerse yourself in the practices outlined in the protocol & make yog a way of life. By doing so, you will embark on a transformative journey that not only reduces your physical fat but also nurtures your five layers of personality, all while fostering healthier dietary habits. I extend my blessings to this creation.

Yog brings changes in the thinking of person & also develops the tolerance in an individual

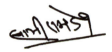

Dr. H.R. Nagendra - Guruji

Chancellor of S-Vyasa University.

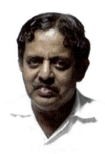

In the pursuit of health and happiness, we encounter two paths
– *Sukh Praptihih (happiness) and Dukhah Nivrittihih (suffering).*

The science of 'Yog' embodies one such stream of knowledge, offering a time-tested, scientific approach to solving many problems in human life. Among the challenges we face today, childhood obesity stands as a major health concern that requires urgent attention and effective solutions. It is our collective responsibility to support our young generation in overcoming this obstacle and paving the way for a healthier future. Constructive measures must be taken to address this pressing issue, and 'Yog' emerges as a promising solution. I am delighted to learn that my esteemed student, Dr. Sunanda Rathi, who completed her doctoral research under my guidance, has undertaken the noble cause of combating childhood obesity through the path of 'Yog.' As a Ph.D. candidate at S-Vyasa University, she has exemplified dedication and passion in her pursuit of knowledge and service.I am confident that this book will serve as an effective tool in the ongoing battle against the global problem of childhood obesity and the related health issues it brings. Dr. Sunanda's meticulous efforts and dedication to this noble cause are commendable, and I extend my heartfelt blessings to her. May we, through concerted efforts and the wisdom of 'Yog,' triumph in our mission to establish global health and well-being.

Let us embrace the path of 'Yog' and empower our younger generation to lead healthier, happier lives.

Dr. R. Nagarathna - Didi

MD, MRCP, FRCP Dean of the Division of Yoga and Life Sciences at Arogyadhama, S-Vyasa.

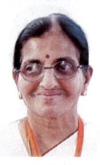

Obesity has become one of the most common and costly chronic disorders globally, affecting individuals of all genders and age groups. It is not merely a passive accumulation of excess weight but involves a deeper imbalance within the body. Dr. Sunanda's book takes a holistic approach, centered around the practice of Yoga, to introduce lifestyle changes to children and adolescents struggling with obesity. Research has shown that obese adolescents are at a higher risk of developing multiple physical and psychological complications, such as insulin resistance, dyslipidemia, type 2 diabetes mellitus, hypertension, polycystic ovarian syndrome, metabolic syndrome, and more, in their adulthood. By addressing obesity in its early stages, we can prevent and manage these serious health conditions. I am pleased to see that this book not only focuses on the individual but also emphasizes the importance of family and community involvement in tackling childhood obesity. Parents and teachers play a crucial role in creating a healthy environment at home and school, promoting regular yoga and physical exercise, adopting better dietary practices, and encouraging a vibrant and non-sedentary lifestyle. Obesity may have a genetic predisposition, but it is also influenced by our plate – what we eat – and our lifestyle choices. By adopting the practices and insights shared in this book by co-author Aashish S Rathi for children, parents, and the entire community can embrace a healthier way of living.

I wholeheartedly recommend this book to parents, teachers, and all those concerned about the health and future of our younger generation.

RNagarathna

Mentor Shri. Ramkumar Rathi

Yog Sadhak - Yog Promotor

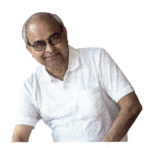

In today's fast-paced and technology-driven world, childhood obesity has emerged as a pressing concern that demands our immediate attention. As we witness a rising tide of health issues among our younger generation, it is essential to take proactive steps to safeguard their well-being and pave the way for a healthier future. I am delighted & honored to pen this forward for " Reduce – A Guide to Prevent Childhood Obesity," a remarkable book by Dr Sunanda Rathi. With great expertise & passion, she has crafted a comprehensive guide to combat childhood obesity through the powerful combination of yoga and mindful eating habits. In the pages that follow, readers will find a wealth of scientific knowledge, practical advice, and actionable insights. Her commitment to promote holistic health shines through as they present a well researched and evidence-based approach to address the challenges of child and adolescent obesity. What sets this book apart is its emphasis on the transformative power of yoga, not just as a physical exercise but as a life-changing practice that nurtures the mind, body, & soul. Throughout my career in the field of health and wellness, I have witnessed the immense impact that holistic practices like yoga can have on an individual's life. It gives me immense joy to see an author championing the cause of healthier living for the younger generation. I extend my heartfelt appreciation to Dr Sunanda & Aashish for their dedication, research, and commitment to creating a healthier world for our children.

I encourage readers to embark on this transformative journey with an open mind and a willingness to embrace positive change.

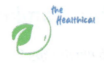

Testimonial
Dr. Sanjay Malpani

Founder Chairman- Dhruv Global School

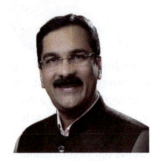

Dr. Sanjay Malpani is President of Asian Yogasana & Vice President of World Yogasana. He is Vice President of Yogasana Bharat & President of Maharashtra Yogasana Sport Association. He is industrialist & Academician holds the position as the President of Brihan Maharashtra Yoga Parishad & Chairman of Madhavlal Malpani Naturopathy & Yoga Centre.

I personally and on behalf of students and parents of Dhruv School expressed thanks for choosing Dhruv School for the study project by Dr Sunanda Rathi

I am extremely pleased to share my experiences with Chiranjiv Foundation and Dr. Sunanda Rathi, as the Founder Chairman of Dhruv Global School. Dr. Rathi and her team conducted a one month yoga protocol for our students and teachers, introducing us to their innovative protocol. This initiative began as a pilot project, and the impact it had was truly remarkable.

Dr. Rathi explained the entire protocol to us, outlining how it would work and what we could expect. We decided to implement this protocol in our Obese students, and the results were astounding. Within the very first week, we began to witness positive changes in the students who were part of the program.

By incorporating the yoga protocol and promoting healthy eating habits, we observed significant improvements in the children's overall well-being. Notably, there was a substantial reduction in their weight, accompanied by improvements in mood, energy levels, and concentration. In just 30 days, on average, we witnessed a remarkable 5 to 8 kilograms of weight loss in the participating students.

What truly warmed our hearts was the collective happiness of both parents and teachers. The positive changes were not limited to physical aspects but also transcended into other facets of the students' lives, including their academic performance and emotional well-being. Additionally, we were pleasantly surprised by the changes reflected in the student's blood reports, which indicated a healthier, more balanced state.

Based on our experience, I wholeheartedly recommend implementing this protocol in all schools, and I believe it should also be embraced by parents and teachers alike. The benefits we observed were not merely superficial; they contributed significantly to the overall growth and development of the children. Dr. Sunanda Rathi and the Chiranjiv Foundation have provided us with an invaluable tool for the betterment of our students' lives, and I am grateful for the positive impact it has had on our school community.

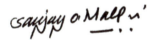

"Embrace the Yoga Protocol, Transform Your Life. For Obese Students, it's the path to Reduce & Balance your weight for Concerned Parents, it's the key to Health & Harmony; and for Dedicated Teachers, it's the source of Strength & Serenity. Make Yoga Your Lifestyle, Gift Yourself Wellness, and reverse Obesity.

Acknowledgement

The hardest part of the book is to pen down in these allotted pages;it is just an impossible task. The success and final outcome of this book have required a lot of guidance and assistance from many people and I am extremely privileged to have that. There is a bridge between my research and its publication in the form of a book that only knows those who have helped me to cross the same. I will not forget to express it. If words are considered to be signs of gratitude, then let these words convey the very same, My utmost sincere gratitude to all the eminent professionals whose whole hearted support and contribution have made this book possible.

First and foremost, my intellectual debt is to those yog academicians and yog practitioners who have contributed significantly to the emerging field of yogic processes and practices and whose work has been quoted significantly and used extensively in writing this book.

Firstly, I thank the Lord Almighty for the abundant grace in my life, for giving me an opportunity to undertake this project and for his grace in seeing its completion. I wish to convey my sincere gratitude to University S-Vyasa, an esteemed and sacred Institution, to have given me a divine opportunity to learn this ancient wonderful wisdom of YOG.

I express my respectful gratitude to Padma Shri Dr H.R. Nagendra. Whatever I learned about this journey is because of his guidance. His support throughout my research period was unimaginable and encouraging. Only because of his inspiration, suggestions and care, I stand where I am today. I am grateful to him for giving me an opportunity to work with him and for his trust in my abilities. I express my gratitude to Dr. Padmini Tekur for her constant guidance, support and encouragement. I owe my heartfelt gratitude to Dr R. Nagarathna, Medical Director, S-Vyasa for all the support & valuable suggestions.

Very special heartfelt gratitude to my mentor Mr. Ramkumarji Rathi. I am grateful to him and fortunate enough to get his constant encouragement and inspiration without which this book would not have taken off. My academic colleagues at S-Vyasa University deserve my appreciation for extending to me their wholehearted cooperation and support. I would be doing an injustice if I forget to convey my gratitude to Dr. Sanjay Malpani, Chairman of Dhruv School, who let me use the campus of Dhruv School, a residential school at Sangamner, Maharashtra for my pilot study during my Ph.D. Big thanks to the Principal and staff for providing support to students who participated in the study. I am extremely thankful to Smt. Malti Kalmadi of Kaveri Education, Pune for permitting us to conduct our main study at Dr. Shamrao Kalmadi School in Pune and to the principal and staff for their help for pre- and post-data collection for the main study and conduction of our intervention in the school premises.

I am extremely grateful to my friends, yoga consultants and eminent scholars for extending their immense contribution and support in writing the text script of this book and for providing me with their utmost guidance on this specific subject, which is really very important content in this book. I have learned a lot from my parents and especially from my late father, who was my first "Guru" who taught me the importance of education, self-study, values, and ethics. I am grateful to my husband Dr. Surendra Rathi and my mother Smt. Leeladevi, who has provided me with moral and emotional support in my life. I am also grateful to my children and family members, friends, and well-wishers for their great support and strength.

I will always remain thankful to my staff of Chiranjiv Foundation & Arena Animation Tilak Road, Pune. I am indebted to the Chiranjeev Animation Studio for the efforts they have put in for the creative design for this book and the 3D models created for yoga postures & to Nitesh Paikrao for layout of the book. I owe my gratitude to Beeja Publication, Geetika Saigal & her team. Let us end with you, the readers. Thanks for not only buying a copy, and reading it, but practicing the yoga protocol and promoting the same to all obese and overweight friends and relatives, however, I would, further, welcome any suggestion for making the next edition of this book more useful to the readers.

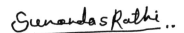

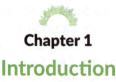

Chapter 1

Introduction

*"You must keep a strict eye on your health;
let everything else be subordinated to that."*
Swami Vivekanand

"Trust me, I've been trying everything to lure him out of the house but nothing works out. He even finds excuses to skip school these days." Pallavi, a family friend, was complaining about her 14-year old son, Reyan. It was a birthday party and I had casually asked her how Reyan missed a chance to have his favorite cake. I had opened Pandora's box. Soon I realized that what appeared to be casual complaining, had much more gravity. It didn't seem like the usual 'teenage rebellion' case. Reyan was going to great lengths to avoid his peers and people in general. After getting to know more about his behavioral pattern, I realized that he may be suffering from some psychological disorder. Before concluding anything, I had to meet him once in person. To avoid any more excuses from him, we came up with a plan to catch him off guard.

Next Sunday, I arrived at Pallavi's place early in the morning. Both Pallavi and Avinash, the worried parents were home and acted as surprised as planned. After multiple trips by his parents to his room, Reyan came out and sat in front of me. His reluctance was evident in his 'Namaste!' with the slightest smile possible.

"Hello, Reyan!" I replied. I was meeting him after at least a year and a half and the change in his appearance was significant. It wasn't just his age. For such a short period, he had put on a substantial amount of weight. He was walking slowly and had visible stretch marks around his arms and calf areas. The dark patches on the neck were even indicating high sugar levels. Reyan had always been a healthy child with some baby fat on the cheeks, but I was quite shocked to see him visibly obese. After the initial small talk, Pallavi eagerly wanted to shift the conversation to Reyan. But he was smart enough to realize that my early morning visit may not be by chance.

"It all started after his bicycle accident because of his fractured leg. He lost one whole academic year and had to take rest for a long time. Even after the treatment, he was advised not to put pressure on the injured leg. so he turned to computer games and that's when it all escalated. It has become quite a task to take him away from these gadgets. I think his friends have also started avoiding him due to this!"

"Who told you that they're the ones to avoid me? It was 'me', who chose not to be with them, okay? All they want to do is bully me and talk nonsense about how I resemble a cow. Why do you still want me to be friends with them?" Pallavi was promptly interrupted by Reyan. The distressed mother was surprised at his loud outburst. I intervened as she started scolding him for not behaving. I asked Reyan if he'd like to take a walk with me. Reluctantly, he agreed. Probably to try to escape from his mother's wrath. During the short walk in their housing society's park, I tried to get to the root cause of the situation. Reyan had seen me often since he was a baby. Fortunately, he trusted me enough to open up about his stress and insecurities.

My doubts about his disturbing psychological health were confirmed. He was showing the early signs of depression. A condition that is disturbingly common these days among teens. In the case of Reyan, his journey towards depression was just a by-product of a much more severe problem. 'Obesity in Children and Adolescents' is one of the most serious health issues that are prevalent today. Not just in India but the entire world is battling this growing societal health problem, and it demands much more attention than it's currently receiving. The issue is grave, especially in the urban parts of the world. It's the biggest catalyst in the increasing burden of diseases worldwide. Mental as well as physical.

This 'New World Syndrome', called 'Obesity' has been equally rampant in developed, developing as well as under-developed countries, causing a major socio-economic and public health concern. Obesity occurs due to overeating, having junk food or nutrient-poor food, and living a sedentary lifestyle. In the case of children, parents have to recognize this as a serious issue at the appropriate age and time, to prevent various morbidities caused by obesity, such as the increased risk of diabetes, hypertension, heart disease, sleep apnea, and cancer. Obesity not just affects the physical well-being of a person but sometimes it may even hamper psychological health as many parts of society stigmatize obesity. This can result in alienation of the obese children due to less socialization. It further increases the chances of psychological comorbidities like depression.

This is exactly what happened with Reyan. The initial immobility due to his accident led to prolonged inactivity and lethargy which was also fueled by his exposure to video games and long hours on the internet. His insecurities about his appearance and the constant bullying by his peers about the same further drifted him apart. Lastly, he was burdened by his parents to maintain his grades and status in school. The poor child couldn't take it anymore and his mental health had taken a toll. His grades had worsened as a result, making it a vicious cycle.

Reyan's case is not a unique phenomenon. Today's generation has everything in abundance. Life has become more comfortable than ever before. The extent of exposure and opportunities that are available to this generation, give them access to various experiences in life at least a decade earlier than their parents received it. Everything seems to be practically preponed for them. This rush to live early, the rush to have everything early turns life into a race. Hence comes the compulsion to win. And to win a race, one has to touch the finish line at the earliest. Does this not mean that you are essentially trying to 'finish' the race of life early? Does that really make you a winner?

The fast-paced life poses new challenges every day not just for adults but also for children. They are expected to prove their potential in every field, resulting in negligence towards the most important front of their life, their physical, mental, and emotional health. Therefore, the first thing you need to understand is that life is not a race to finish in a hurry. It's a journey to experience and enjoy. And to be able to fully indulge in it, we have to be completely healthy. Physically, as well as mentally. This is why it is important to prevent obesity at the early stage of life. Except for medical conditions such as hormonal imbalance, the most common causes of obesity among children are the lack of physical activity, unhealthy eating patterns, or a combination of these factors.I had learned about Reyan's overall daily routine which did not include physical exercises of any form. Apparently, he didn't like to indulge in sports or school gym to stay away from some of his peers. He poured his heart out to me about his traumatic experience with the bullies and I supported his decision to avoid them.

I casually asked him if he had ever heard of 'yoga asanas. He remembered doing Surya Namaskar in school at some point but never pursuing it thereafter. I told him how yoga asanas can be one way of maintaining his physical fitness even while being at home. He seemed intrigued. While returning home, I slipped some more interesting facts about yoga to him. By the time we reached, he even started asking a question or two. Pallavi and Avinash seemed relieved to see him engaged in a conversation with someone. Soon, they joined in and I introduced them to the familiar yet unexplored world of yoga.

'Yog!' This artistic and scientific approach toward life deals with the evolution of the mind and body. It includes all aspects of human existence, from physical health to self-realization.

A child is supposed to be the most open-minded of all human beings. This open mind is intuitive, creative and has tremendous potential to learn new things. Hence, the ideal time to inculcate Yoga Practice in a person is childhood, so that it can lead to balanced and healthy adulthood.

I had been working in the field of 'Yog for Children' for quite some time now. This helped me understand Reyan's case better. During my research tour for bringing awareness about childhood obesity, I was once invited to a residential school in Maharashtra. During my visit, I came across various obesity-related health issues in children including PCOD, stress, and depression. When we implemented a yoga program for these students, a lot of them experienced immediate positive effects. When they continued the practice of yoga asanas, most of their long-term health complaints related to excessive weight disappeared. This motivated me to help spread this amazing science amongst as many youngsters as I could.

Chapter 2
Obesity as per Ancient Indian Literature

QUICK START

According to the ancient Indian scriptures, to bring about a balance, "samatolanam", at the physical level, a person has to be treated as a whole, body and mind. We should start tackling this problem from a philosophical point of view

The call to embrace a healthy lifestyle through mindful eating finds its roots in ancient wisdom, echoing the teachings of our scriptures. The Bhagavad Gita, a revered ancient text, provides profound insights and recommendations on healthy living. Additionally, Ayurveda, the Science of Life, represents the empirical knowledge amassed over 5000 years in India. Timeless texts like Charak Sahita and Madhav Nidan stand as testaments to this rich tradition, encapsulating the holistic approach to well-being advocated by our ancestors.

Obesity is described as one of the eight types of undesirable constitutions in Charaka Samhitā by Charaka, the great ancient scholar of Ayurveda, stated that people who are Atisthula (overweight) are more likely to be at a health risk than those who are at a normal weight.

In Chapter 21, Volume 1 of Charaka Samhitā, it is mentioned that obese people have a shorter life span; they are physically weak and slow, excessively hungry, thirsty and emit bad smells.

In Charak Samhita, one of the foundational texts of Ayurveda, obesity is described as a condition primarily caused by an imbalance in the Kapha dosha. According to Ayurvedic principles, Kapha governs the structure and lubrication in the body. When Kapha is aggravated due to factors such as improper diet, lack of physical activity, and sedentary lifestyle, it leads to an accumulation of excess fat tissues, causing obesity. Charak Samhita emphasizes the significance of balanced digestion and metabolism. When digestion is weak, it leads to the formation of ama (undigested toxins), contributing to weight gain. Additionally, emotional factors such as stress, anxiety, and depression are believed to disrupt the balance of doshas and contribute to obesity.

The text prescribes a holistic approach to tackle obesity, including dietary modifications, physical exercises, herbal treatments, and lifestyle changes. It emphasizes the importance of a balanced and wholesome diet, regular exercise, and maintaining emotional well-being to prevent and manage obesity effectively.

Madhav Nidan, an ancient text in Ayurveda, delves into the intricate understanding of obesity and its causes. According to this revered scripture, obesity is attributed to an imbalance in the body doshas, particularly Kapha dosha. The accumulation of ama (toxins) due to improper digestion and metabolism is considered a primary cause. Additionally, sedentary lifestyle, excessive consumption of sweet, fatty, and oily foods, lack of physical activity, and emotional imbalances are outlined as major factors leading to obesity in Madhav Nidan. This holistic perspective emphasizes the importance of balancing one's lifestyle, diet, and emotional well-being to prevent and manage obesity.

Causes & Effects Of Obesity

	OBESITY	
01 Physical inactivity / Sedentary lifestyle		Insulin resistance / Diabetes
02 Environments		Cadio Vascular Disease (CVD)
03 Genetics		Arthtitis
04 Socio econimics status		Cancer
05 Eating behaviour / Over-eating poor nutrients		Infertility

Chapter 3
Etiology of Obesity: Causes
(Based on Research Study)

KICK START

The current obesity epidemic is due to societal changes involving both physical activity and food consumption patterns and cultural changes.

Eating Habits & Physical Activities:

All weight loss programs need a change in eating habits, diet, what to eat and what not to eat and increased physical activities.

The maintenance of the reduced body weight is much more difficult for the obese as they eventually return to their initial body weight and in most cases even heavier than before. Prevention of weight gain seems to be the general strategy to tackle obesity. Most food plans for weight loss emphasize providing age-appropriate food portion sizes, reducing fast food meals, increasing fruits and vegetable consumption and structured meal times.

The study indicates that fiber-rich diets containing non-starchy vegetables, fruits, whole grains, legumes, and nuts may be effective in the prevention and treatment of obesity in child primary school children's physical fitness is associated with their eating habits and decreases the number of unhealthy eating behaviors cumulated (Thivel, Tremblay, & Chaput, 2013).

In another study, it is observed that in obesity reduction, regular physical activity has been traditionally considered as a strategy to burn calories and a stimulus if properly managed, contributes to a significant improvement of energy and macronutrient balance regulation and body functionality. Effective long-term weight loss depends on permanent changes in dietary quality, energy intake, and activity. Neither medical management nor societal preventive challenges are currently being met (Haslam & James, 2005).

Genetic Factors in Obesity:
Several studies have shown that there is a strong genetic basis for the development of obesity. It appears to be a polygenic disorder, with many genes currently linked or associated with a predisposition to excess adiposity. Overweight and obesity represent an increasing health problem. Both genetic and environmental factors contribute to the development of obesity. The genetic influence on body weight is shown by twin and family studies. Environmental changes in recent decades have promoted the development of obesity in individuals at risk because of their genetic composition.

As per the study of Qi & Cho, understanding of the molecular pathways underlying common obesity is limited. During the last decade, a handful of monogenic disorders leading to early, severe obesity in humans have been identified. All affect the central regulation of appetite. Knowledge of genetic and environmental components may facilitate the choice of more effective and specific measures for obesity prevention based on the personalized genetic makeup (Qi & Cho, 2008).

Sedentary Behaviors:
Research studies indicate that Sedentary life with little physical activity is the major lifestyle change in modern fast life that contributes to the increasing prevalence of obesity. Sedentary lifestyle patterns in children and adolescents, playing digital games, using computers and watching television, have been associated with obesity. A review including published studies found in PubMed and other medical journals, dated between January 1990 and April 2007. The age between 2-18 years of children and adolescents who were the object of the study, selected cross-sectional, longitudinal and intervention studies, video games and computers, and watching TV, represent a high risk when they do not replace physical activity too much (Rey-López, Vicente Rodríguez, Biosca, & Moreno, 2008).

Dietary Intake:
Consumption of high-calorie foods with little spending time for burning, results in the accumulation of the surplus energy that gets accumulated in fat cells. Dietary intake throughout childhood is a key factor in growth and development and plays an important role in the prevention and treatment of childhood overweight and obesity.

The review by Collins, Watson on current dietary intake assessment methodologies for children, provides guidance on how these can be improved reporting of dietary intakes of overweight children in the literature and identify future research priorities (Collins, Watson, & Burrows, 2010).

Parental Obesity, Eating Patterns and Attitudes:
Parental obesity more than doubles the risk of adult obesity among both obese and non-obese children. Bad dietary habits of the mother of preschoolers are associated with subsequent excess weight gain in their daughters. The intensity of parental involvement and behavior change techniques are important issues in the effectiveness of long-term childhood weight control interventions (Van Der Kruk, Kortekaas, Lucas, & Jager-Wittenaar, 2013)

Obesity is the most prevalent form of malnutrition. It is prevalent in both developed and underdeveloped countries. Obesity happens at any age. One of the causes of obesity is that the amount of abdominal fat is influenced by the genetic compound physical inactivity; not performing physical work leads to obesity. Psychological factors; anxiety, worries, and loneliness also leads to obesity. Environmental labor-saving devices such as escalators and lifts, computer games and fewer manual occupations have led to a reduction in physical activity levels. People who have obesity, compared to those with a normal or healthy weight, are at increased risk for many serious diseases and health conditions, including the following:

- All causes of death (mortality)
- High blood pressure (Hypertension)
- High LDL cholesterol, low HDL cholesterol, or high levels of triglycerides (Dyslipidemia)
- Type 2 diabetes
- Coronary heart disease
- Stroke
- Gallbladder disease
- Osteoarthritis - a breakdown of cartilage and bone within a joint
- Sleep apnea and breathing problems

"Childhood obesity isn't some simple, discrete issue. There's no one cause that we can pinpoint. There's no one program we can fund to make it go away. Rather, it's an issue that touches on every aspect of how we live and how we work."

– Michelle Obama

Yog helps in maintaining command over one's own mind, body, and soul. It's a beautiful amalgamation of physical and mental disciplines to achieve peace of body and mind. It assists you in managing stress and anxiety and keeps you relaxed. Regular practice of yog helps maintain physical health by increasing flexibility, muscle strength, and body tone.

The younger generation is, and always has been the most important factor in shaping society. By helping them to attain holistic well-being, Yog can be the much-needed catalyst to create a better future for them and for the generations to come.

After we discussed how yog can help improve the overall physical and mental health of a person and hence the family, both Pallavi and Avinash strongly felt that they need to include this rejuvenating habit into their lifestyle. Even Reyan agreed to give it a try. A small but promising step indeed. We immediately began the implementation and soon it started producing the fruits of success.

Parental support is also a crucial element in this journey. The problem of obesity must be detected and accepted early by parents so that they can help their children in overcoming the same. A lot of parents believe that obesity is genetic or hereditary and no external intervention can help. Though a genetic factor can be present, it is observed that most of the cases are due to the problem of over-eating, or consumption of non-nutritious junk food. Excessive screen time and a sedentary lifestyle add to this. All of these can be prevented with some parental control. Additionally, when obesity starts affecting the mental health of children, they need parental care and affection to cope with it. I would like to mention that Pallavi and Avinash went to great lengths to understand the roots of their child's depression and helped him come out of it in as many ways as they could.

This whole ordeal provoked me to speed up the process of bringing this book into the world. My encounter with the students of many schools in Maharashtra who were fighting various obesity related issues had already planted a seed in my mind about this book. I realized how much effort is still needed to be put in order to help spread the ancient wisdom of yog for the betterment of the younger generation.

In this project, we aim to make yog fun and engaging for children and youngsters so that they not just learn but continue to practice it for life. Keeping this in mind, we have designed a yoga intervention.

The purpose of this book, 'Reduce – A Guide to Prevent Childhood Obesity" is to present the knowledge of scientific yog practices to help conquer the problem of obesity globally. It aims to provide scientific research-based yog protocol and an Integrated Approach to Yog Therapy (IAYT) for 'Child & Adolescent Obesity. This protocol is a preventive measure against child & adolescent obesity and has been already validated and implemented on school-going children of Maharashtra showing tremendous results in fat and weight reduction.

> *"Yoga becomes the destroyer of pain for those who are moderate in eating and recreation (such as walking, etc.), who are moderate in exertion in actions, who are moderate in sleep and wakefulness." - Bhagavad Gita Chapter 6 Verse 17*
> *(Translated by Swami Vivekananda)*

I hope this book helps many more children like Reyan and also their parents, to understand how they can have control over their physical and psychological health through Yog.

Chapter 4
What is Yog & its Benefits in Daily Life

KICK START

*"How do you ensure your well-being and sustained vitality?
The answer lies in yog, the art and science of wholesome living."*

Definition of Yog:
Yog, as defined in Patanjali's Yoga Sutras, 1.2,
"Yogas citta-vrtti-nirodhah."
This definition is from a foundational text in the philosophy and practice of yog.
Translation: "Yog is the restraint of the modifications of the mind." In this context, "citta" refers to the mind, "vrtti" to the fluctuations or modifications of the mind, and "nirodhah" to the restraint or control. The ultimate goal of yog, as described in this sutra and throughout the Yog Sutras, is to achieve a state of inner peace, clarity, and self-realization by quieting the constant chatter and distractions of the mind.

In other Defination: Yog-Vasishta says
"manah prashamanah yog ityabhidhiyate" which means that yog is a skillful method to calm the mind.

Yog is the most precious gift to mankind for a healthy life. It is about a 5000-year-old Indian philosophy that combines exercise, breathing, diet, relaxation and meditation developed by our elderly spiritual saints and sages. The subject of yog has been dealt with extensively in many ancient Indian scriptures like – Patanjali Yog Sutras, Bhagavad Gita, Upanishads, Yog Vasishta, Hatha Yog Pradipika, Gheranda Samhita, Siva Samhita, Puranas, etc. Also in recent times, eminent spiritual leaders like Swami Vivekananda and Sri Aurobindo have further clarified the concept and purpose of Yog philosophy. The efforts of our Honorable Prime Minister Shri Narendra Modi in spreading and creating awareness of Yog and its benefits is seen as we now celebrate the International Yog Day all over the world on 21st June.

Benefits of doing Yog:

Yog can offer numerous benefits to children, both physically and mentally. Introducing yog into a child's routine can help improve their overall well-being and development. Here are some of the benefits of doing yog for kids:

1. Physical Health:

    a. Flexibility: Yog postures (asanas) can enhance a child's flexibility, helping to prevent injuries and improve posture.
    b. Strength: Yog poses can build core strength, balance, and muscle tone.
    c. Coordination: Practicing yog encourages better coordination and body awareness.
    d. Endurance: Regular yog practice can boost a child's stamina and energy levels.

2. Mental Health:

    a. Stress Reduction: Yog teaches relaxation techniques and deep breathing, which can help kids manage stress and anxiety.
    b. Emotional Regulation: Children can learn to better control their emotions and reactions through mindfulness and self-awareness.
    c. Concentration: Yog promotes focus and concentration, which can aid in schoolwork and other activities.
    d. Self-Esteem: Achieving yog poses can boost a child's self-confidence and sense of accomplishment.
    e. Mindfulness: Yog encourages being present in the moment, which can lead to greater awareness and appreciation of life.

3. Emotional and Social Development:

    a. Empathy: Yog can foster empathy and kindness by teaching kids to respect their own and others' bodies and feelings.
    b. Communication: Practicing partner or group yog poses can improve communication and teamwork skills.
    c. Stress Management: Yog can help children cope with challenging situations and transitions in life.

d. Emotional Resilience: Yog can equip kids with tools to deal with setbacks and difficulties.

4. Better Sleep:
A regular yog practice can lead to improved sleep patterns and better sleep quality, which is crucial for a child's growth and development.

5. Body Awareness:
Yog helps children connect with and appreciate their bodies, leading to healthier habits and a positive body image.

6. Enhanced Breathing:
Yog teaches kids to breathe deeply and mindfully, which can improve lung capacity and respiratory health.

7. Creativity:
Yog encourages creativity and imagination through story-telling, visualization, and imaginative play within yoga poses.

8. Mind-Body Connection:
Yog fosters an understanding of the interconnectedness of the body, mind, and spirit.

9. Fun and Playfulness:
Yog can be made fun and engaging for kids through playful activities and games, making it an enjoyable way to stay active.

10. Non-Competitive:
Yog is non-competitive, allowing children to progress at their own pace and build self-acceptance.

11. Spiritual Enlightenment:
The pursuit of spiritual enlightenment is at the core of yogic philosophy. Through self-reflection, introspection, and a deepening awareness of one's inner self, individuals can transcend the boundaries of the ego and connect with a higher, universal consciousness. This spiritual journey often leads to a profound sense of purpose, inner fulfillment, and a deep connection with the universe and all living beings.

It's important to note that children should be guided by qualified yog instructors or educators who are experienced in teaching yog to kids. Yog for kids often incorporates games, stories, and age-appropriate techniques to make it engaging and enjoyable. Overall, yog can be a valuable tool for promoting physical and mental well-being in children and helping them develop life skills that will serve them throughout their lives.

So yog is a transformative journey that goes beyond physical postures. Yog is not just a tool for weight loss; it is a profound philosophy and a way of life that encompasses much more than physical fitness. While yog can certainly aid in achieving a healthy body weight, its benefits extend far beyond the physical realm.

The commitment to regular practice cultivates self-discipline, leading to positive lifestyle changes and improved overall health. The structured nature of yog practice encourages individuals to stay dedicated and focused, paving the way for personal growth and transformation.

It is crucial to understand that yog is not a quick fix or a temporary solution. It is a lifelong journey that requires dedication, discipline, and continuous practice. While weight loss and physical fitness might be initial motivations for many practitioners, the true essence of yog lies in its ability to bring about inner peace, mental clarity, and spiritual growth.

So, dear reader, as you embark on your yog journey, remember that it is not just about shedding pounds but about gaining a deeper understanding of yourself, cultivating inner harmony, and embracing a holistic approach to life. May your yog practice bring you not only a healthy body but also a peaceful mind and a joyful spirit.

Let us deep dive into yog...Are you ready to move ahead & make yog your lifestyle.

Sage Patanjali in 1.14 sutra of Samadhi Pada says

sa tu dirghakalanairantaryasatkarasevito dridha-bhoomih

It (Abhyasa) becomes firmly grounded by long constant efforts, uninterruptedly, with earnest devotion.

Chapter 5

Integrated Approach of Yog Therapy

(Yog Protocol for Obesity)

KICK START

I remembered a discussion with Reyan, who expressed with agony that I am labeled as obese. When you put a label on someone, the label becomes his limitation. Friends, parents, teachers and society have to be very careful about their external words as they quickly become the child's internal words.

The yog protocol outlined in this chapter offers research-based solutions, providing a holistic approach to obesity without any side effects. Grounded in scientific research and ancient wisdom, these practices offer a comprehensive solution to tackle obesity, focusing on physical, mental, and emotional well-being. By embracing this protocol, individuals can achieve lasting results and improve their overall health without the risks associated with other methods. It stands as a testament to the power of holistic and natural approaches in managing and preventing obesity.

Why is a sequence so important in yog practices? What is to be done?

A yog protocol which is developed by me, Dr Rathi with the help of experts and validated and introduced in the schools as the research study begins with the practice of physical body postures or asanas - which helps to maintain the spinal column, muscles and joints in a healthy state and also helps in the proper functioning of various glands and reducing fats. It has a wide range of physical benefits which include maintaining a correct posture and boosting the functioning of the nervous system, digestive system, and respiratory system. Further practice includes breathing techniques and pranayama - which help in the proper functioning of the lungs and also have a direct effect on the brain and emotional stability.

Meditation practices incorporated influenced weight loss. Lower levels of uncontrolled eating were associated with meditation practices. Meditation helped reduce dysfunctional eating behaviors. Anxiety levels were reduced by meditation practices. Overweight children who meditated had shown satisfactory effects on eating behavior. It involves relaxation or pratyahara by withdrawing from external distractions and concentrating on oneself, which helps reduce stress and results in a reduction of adipose tissues and abdominal fats.

The psychological benefits include relieving stress from day-to-day life, maintaining emotional stability, increasing the capacity to concentrate and remember, improving imagination, visualization and developing one's personality. Inculcating yoga practices right from a young age and encouraging children to adopt them as a lifestyle will help them reap the maximum of these benefits. It can also help in channelsing the energy in the right direction and improving concentration for hyperactive and aggressive children. Emotionally disturbed children can also benefit from practicing yoga. There have been successful cases of practicing yoga protocol for obesity being helpful for PCOD.

Childhood obesity is an issue of serious medical and social concern due to the adoption of a western lifestyle. Consumption of high-calorie food, lack of physical activity and increased time on television are major risk factors for childhood obesity. Obese adolescents are more prone to adopt the risk of medical and psychological complications like Insulin resistance, dyslipidemia, type 2 diabetes mellitus, hypertension, polycystic ovarian syndrome and metabolic syndrome in their adulthood. Prevention and treatment of obesity involves lifestyle modification of the entire family.

Note: The time of practicing this protocol has to be adjusted as per the availability at disposal but it is suggested to practice in the early morning in fresh air. Performing in the sequence is essential. We can select from loosening on an alternate basis like in Yogasana of Standing, sitting, prone & supine Similarly in breathing techniques. Pranayama Surya Alumon Nadi 27 rounds four times before food is must every day. Daily practice is essential to get the overall benefits.

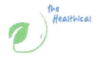

Research Study

Obesity in Adolescents is a worldwide epidemic. Obesity is known to cause heart disease, diabetes, cancer and stroke, the top 4 causes of death. Overeating energy-dense, nutrient-poor foods and a sedentary lifestyle have led to an epidemic of obesity and type 2 diabetes all over the world. It is a global health problem. Apart from physical problems, there are psychological issues which affect the health of the individual. Obesity can be described as a "New World Syndrome" causing an enormous socioeconomic and public health burden in developed, developing and poor countries of the world.

Yog intervention specially designed is known to reduce obesity and enhance psychological well-being. Yog protocol (module specially designed for obesity and validated by Yog experts comprising breathing practices, loosening exercises, asanas (physical postures), pranayama (breathing practices), meditation, devotional sessions and counselling on concepts of the philosophy of Yog like Yogic Counselling and happiness analysis

This Yog Protocol is implemented in two schools:
    1: Residential School   2: Day school

Results: The daily practice of IAYT of 60 minutes in school is useful in managing adolescent obesity. Yog-based intervention is effective to reduce obesity in adolescent children with respect to anthropometric, physical, psychological & cognitive assessments. This study provides evidence to prove the efficacy of Yog to manage increased subcutaneous adiposity in the trunk, hip and leg region resulting in weight reduction in adolescent children. Abdominal circumference is reduced significantly in Yog groups. It is effective in the management of weight, serum triglycerides and very low-density lipoprotein, hip circumference and serum cholesterol. Emotional overeating, enjoyment of food, desire to drink, food fussiness, and satiety responsiveness were reduced in the yog group compared to the control. The perception of bodily awareness has increased in the yog group. In the yog group good concentration, memory and attention were reported. Yog improves emotional well-being in children. Yoga has been reported to have shown beneficial effects on different psychophysiological variables. The yog group has improved better than the control group with an integrated approach to yog therapy.

No.	IAYT SHOWS SCIENTIFIC PROTOCOL OF INTERVENTION	page no	Rounds	Minutes
	PRACTICES			
1.	Opening Prayer	38	1	1
	Yogena Chittasya ----			
2.	**Loosening Exercise: Standing Postures**	39		
A	Jogging: backward, forward & side	40	3	2
B	Jumping	42	3	1
C	Mukha Dhauti	43	1	1/2
D	Backward & Forward Bending	44	10	1
E	Side Bending	45	10	1
F	Spinal Twisting	46	10	1
G	Back Swing	48	5+5	1
H	Hip Rotation	49	5+5	1
I	Hip Stretch	50	5	1
3.	**Surya Namaskara**	51	5+1	6
	Prayer – Hiranmayena Patrena----			
4.	**Yog Asanas**	58		
I	**Standing Postures**	59		
A	Ardha Kati Chakrasana	59	1+1	1
B	Ardha Chakrasana	61	1	1
C	Padahastasana	63	1	1
D	Trikonasana	65	1+1	1
E	Parivrtta Trikonasana	67	1+1	1
II	**Sitting Postures**	69		
A	Vajrasana	69	1	1
B	Ushtrasana	70	1	1
C	Sasankasana	71	1	1
D	Vakrasana	73	1+1	1
E	Spinal Stretch with folded legs	75	1+1	1
F	Bhunamansan	76	5+5	1
G	Chakki Chalana Stretch	77	5+5	1
H	Butterfly	79	10	1
III	**Prone**	80		
A	Bhujangasana	80	1	1

Reduce

No.	IAYT SHOWS SCIENTIFIC PROTOCOL OF INTERVENTION	page no	Rounds	Minutes
	PRACTICES			
B	Parvatasana	82	1	1
C	Dhanurasana	84	1	1
D	Shalabhasana Both legs	85	1+1	1
IV	**Supine**	86	1	1
A	Chakra Padasana (Leg Rotation)	86	5+5	1
B	Pada Sanchalana (Cycling)	87	10	1
C	Chakrasana	89	1	1
D	Setubandhasana	90	1	1
E	Naukasana	92	1	1
5.	**Breathing Practices**	94		
A	Hands In & Out Breathing	95	5	1
B	Hands Stretch Breathing	96	3+3	1
C	Ankle Stretch Breathing	98	5	1
D	Dog Breathing	99	5	1
E	Rabbit Breathing	100	5	1
F	Tiger Breathing	101	5	1
G	Straight Leg Raise Breathing	102		
H	Both Leg Raise	103	5	1
I	Side Leg Raise Breathing	104		
6.	**Kriya-Kapalbhati** **Preparatory Practice for Pranayama**	105	60 to 120	1
7.	**Pranayama**	107		
A	Bhastrika	107		
B	Nadi Shuddhi	109	9	
C	Surya AV 27 rounds 4 times a day	111		
D	Bhramari 9 round	113	9	
8.	**Dhyana**	115		
A	Nadanushandhan	115	9	
B	OM Meditation	117	9	
9.	**Quick Relaxation Technique - QRT**	118		5
10.	**Closing Prayer: Sarve bhavantu Sukhinah**	119	1	1

Reduce

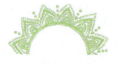

स्थिरसुखमासनम्

Sthira translates as strong, steady, and stable. Sukha means comfortable, happy, and relaxed. Asanam refers to the physical practice of yog. (PS 2-46)

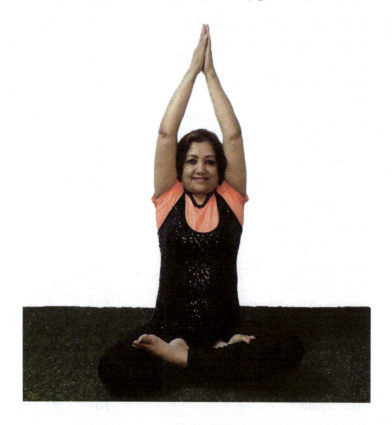

Embark on the transformative journey of practicing this protocol to shed the weight of obesity and regain your vitality. Let this protocol be your guide to a healthier, happier you.

1: Opening Prayer

Why should we start with Prayer? We are in the era of science & technology and we often question everything. We are rational and keen to know why this is so. Research consistently shows that prayer can have numerous benefits. If you pray you can synchronize your mind, body and soul. You are focused on your practices with awareness, breath coordination, and involvement. Prayer can be a solid source of self-soothing and self-comfort. You are cooling yourself down.

Prayer is the act of surrendering oneself to God. It helps a person grow out of his own limitations, helplessness, and a sense of insecurity; thanksgiving, thanking God for his many blessings, e.g., health or children; petition, asking God for something, e.g., healing, courage or wisdom. Prayer is the act of surrendering oneself to God. It helps all to come out of his own limitations, helplessness, and a sense of insecurity. While praying we surrender ourselves to the feet of the Lord realizing that it is the only way to touch the universal consciousness. In the yogic tradition, a prayer has special powers to transform mind, body and spirit.

> "Yogena Cittasya PadenaVacam,
> Malam Sarirasya Ca Vaidyakena,
> YoPakarotam Pravaram Muninam,
> Patanjalim Pranjaliranatosmi,
> Om Santih Santih Santih."

Meaning: I offer my salutations with folded hands to sage Patanjali, the renowned amongst the sages, who removed the impurity of mind through yoga, of speech by grammar, and of body by ayurveda.Om Shanti Shanti !

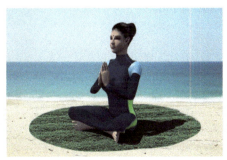

2: Loosening Exercise

KICK OFF

"From childhood, we can train our muscles to support the vertebral joints effectively, thus laying a strong foundation for developing a body with excellent stamina. A flexible and robust spine is considered essential for healthy growth."

This practice helps to flex your spine muscles. Loosen yourself by warming up. Increases blood flow to your muscles and raises your body temperature. This can improve your performance and decrease your risk of injury.

These practices of warm-up help to various joints in the body and increase the flexibility of the spine. Various postures, especially forward bending, twisting, and backward bending, help to reduce fat near the abdomen, hips, and other areas.

Tips

1. Practice the exercises stepwise
2. Count the steps slowly and perform the same with attention
3. Check the performance of each step before increasing the speed
4. Synchronize steps with a group if you are practicing in a group
5. Increase the number of repetitions as per your capacity

Principles

To loosen the various joints in the body.
The flexibility of the spine.

Objectives

Remove lethargy and tiredness in the body.
Build up the stamina of the body.
Discipline the body-mind complex.

A: Jogging

1. Make loose fists of your hands and place them on the chest
2. Collapse and relax your shoulders

Stage 1: Slow Jogging

1. Start Jogging on your toes slowly
2. Jog about 20 to 25 times. As days go by, gradually increase up to 100 times

Stage 2: Backward Jogging

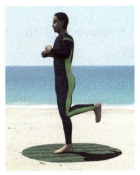

1. Lean a little forward and increase the speed of jogging gradually
2. Start hitting the buttocks with the heels
3. Repeat these 20 -25 times at your maximum speed & capacity
4. Then gradually slow down the speed, do not stop
5. Continue and move on to slow jogging at least 8 to 10 times

Stage 3: Forward Jogging

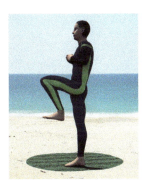

1. Lean backward a little and now as you increase the speed again, try to raise the knees higher and higher
2. Raise the knees forwards to reach the chest level
3. Repeat 20-25 times at your maximum speed and capacity
4. Slow down the practice coming back to the stage of slow jogging again

5. Continue slow jogging for a few rounds, count 10 times

Stage 4: Side Jogging

1. Gradually increase the speed taking the heels sideways

2. As the speed increases bring the heels as much as close to the elbows

3. Repeat this movement 20-25 times at your maximum speed and capacity

4. Gradually slow down to come back to the slow jogging stage

5. Keep jogging a few more rounds 10 to 15 and finally stop the practice

Note:
1. Loose fists and place them on the chest
2. Collapse and relax shoulders
3. Increase the speed of jogging gradually
4. Continue the practice till the 4 stages of jogging
5. Fists on the chest throughout the practice

Benefits:
1. Tones up the calf and thigh muscles
2. Warm up the body
3. Stimulates breathing

"Obesity is not the price children should pay for progress; it's a wake-up call for healthier choices."

B: Jumping

Sthiti: Tadasana

Practice

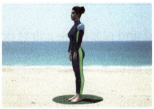

1. Fold the elbows and place the hand with loose fists close to the chest

2. Jump up while touching the heels to the buttocks and then stand on the feet

3. Slowly increase the speed and repeat 10 to 20 times

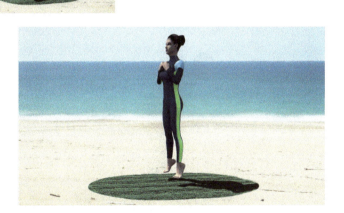

Note:

1. Give good exercise to leg muscles, tones up the calf and thigh muscles

> *"Your body hears everything your mind says keep going. You can!"*

C: Mukha Dhauti To Relax

Sthiti: Tadasana

Practice

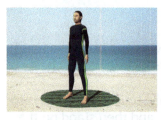

1. Stand erect with legs apart

2. Bend forward and place the palms on the respective thighs keeping the arms and legs straight

3. Inhale through the nose and exhale through the mouth

4. While exhaling blast out the air forcibly through the mouth

5. Then, stand in Tadasana and relax for a while

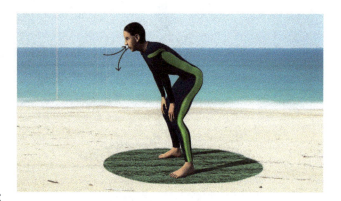

Note:

1. Exhalation in Mukha Dhauti, relieves the strain of jogging and jumping
2. Pulling the abdomen in, during exhalation can improve the force of expulsion of air

> "Raising healthy kids means nourishing their body with love and wholesome choices."

D: Forward And Backward Bending

Sthiti: Tadasana

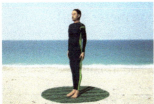

1. Stretch the arms straight above the head with the palm facing forward
2. Inhale & bend backwards with arms stretched above the head
3. While exhaling bend forward as per capacity, do rapidly
4. While bending always bend from the lower waist
5. Easy movements freely and in a flow
6. Repeat 20 to 30 times. Gradually slow down, Stop the practice

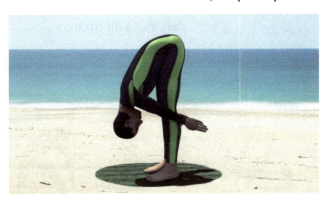

Benefits:

1. Reduces fat from the waist, back, and especially from the abdominal region
2. Increases flexibility of the spine
3. Increases exercise tolerance; helpful in exercise induced asthma
4. Expels blocked air from the lungs
5. Harmonizes the flow of prana
6. Calms down the mind

E: Side Bending

Sthiti: Tadasana

Relax: Sithila Tadasana

Practice

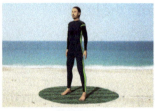

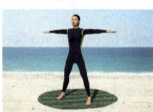

1. Legs about one meter apart
2. Raise the hands sideways parallel to the ground while inhaling
3. Bend to the right till the right-hand touches the right heel while exhaling
4. Look at the palm of the left hand
5. Avoid forward or backward bending
6. Repeat 5 to 6 times to the right and left sides alternately

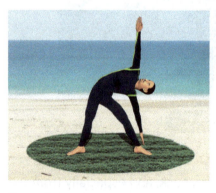
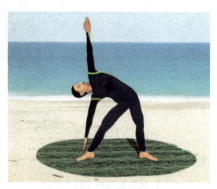

Benefits:

1. Open up the airways of the middle lobes of the lungs
2. Calms down the mind
3. Strengthens the middle part of the chest
4. Empties the middle and upper part of the lungs
5. Stimulates the middle lobe of the lungs

F: Spinal Twisting

Sthiti: Tadasana

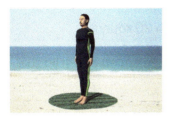

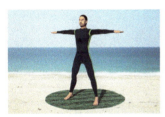

Practice

1. Spread the legs about one meter apart

2. Raise the hands sideways parallel to the ground while inhaling

3. Keep the legs firm on the ground and twist to the right, keeping the right hand straight at shoulder level

4. Simultaneously twist the neck and look at the tip of the fingers. Bend the left hand at the elbow to bring the hand close to the chest

5. Come back while inhaling

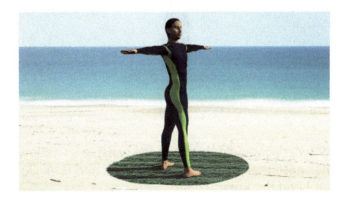

"The best investment we can make in our children's future is to nourish their bodies and minds, not their waistlines."

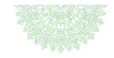

Practice

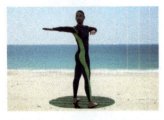

6. Repeat the same on the left

7. Gradually increase the speed to your maximum capacity

8. Repeat 10 to 20 rounds

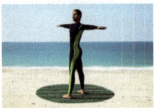

9. Slow down the speed and stop the practice

10. Relax in Tadasana

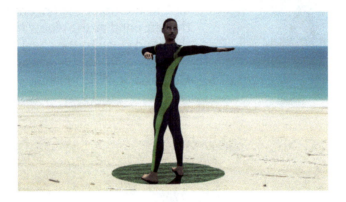

Notes:

All twisting should be above the waist level. Below the waist, maintain the body, straight and firm. Do not bend the knees.

> "The path to a healthy future starts with breaking the chains of childhood obesity."

G: Back Swing
Sthiti: Tadasana

Practice

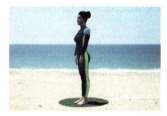

1. Bring the right leg forward with a distance of about one meter between the legs

2. Inhale; simultaneously raise the arms up swinging and arching the back and flexing the knee forward

3. While exhaling, return to Tādāsana

4. Repeat the same with the left leg

5. Practice ten rounds alternately

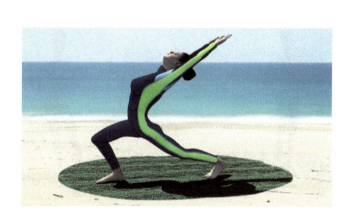

"Childhood obesity doesn't just weigh down the body; it burdens the mind and spirit too."

H: Hip Rotation

Sthiti: Tadasana

Practice

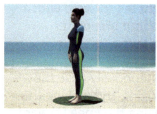

1. Spread the leg about one to two feet apart

2. Place the palms on your waist fingers pointing forwards

3. Start rotating your hip forming a full imaginary circle around your body

4. Keep the knees straight

5. Rotate the hip clockwise and anti-clockwise 10 times each

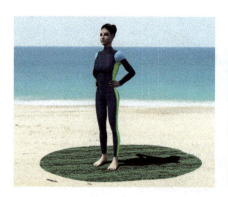
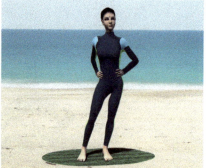

"Childhood obesity is not a fate; it's a challenge we can conquer through determination and compassion."

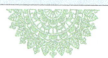

I: Hip Stretch
Sthiti: Tadasana

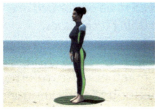

1. Spread the legs apart a little more than a meter

2. Let the feet be parallel to each other

3. Raise the arms forward to shoulder level with palms facing downward

4. Sit on the right foot as you exhale. The left foot is stretched out without bending

5. Come up as you inhale

6. Repeat the practice alternatively 10 times

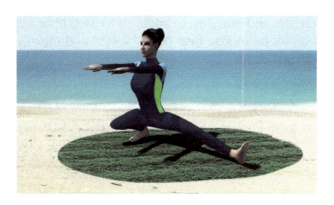

"Fighting childhood obesity is not just a matter of shedding pounds; it's a journey towards self-love and acceptance."

3: Surya Namaskar

KICK OFF

The Surya namaskar can easily be referred to as the father of all the different yoga asanas. Surya Namaskar is a yoga exercise, which is a compilation of 12 different asanas that need to be performed in a certain order with their respective breathing techniques.

This specific detailing of the Surya Namaskar works wonders in bringing the mind, body, and breath together. Also referred to as sun salutation, Surya Namaskar if performed early morning helps keep you energized throughout the day.

Surya namaskar comes in between Loosening Exercise, **'Sithilikarana Vyayama'** and **'Yoga Asanas.'**

It brings about the general flexibility of the body preparing it for Asanas and Pranayama; this is usually done both at sunrise and sunset, facing the Sun.

Surya Namaskar not only promotes weight loss but also strengthens your back, core, and muscles. In addition to metabolic adjustments, Surya namaskar helps you lose belly fat fast and make you get rid of digestion problems.

Prayer

> "Hiranmayena Patrena Satyasyapihitam Mukham
> Tat tvam Pushan Apavrnu Satya Dharmaya Drstaye"
> - Isavasyopanisad

> हिरण्मयेन पात्रेण सत्यस्यापिहितं मुखम्।
> तत्त्वं पूषन्नपावृणु सत्यधर्माय दृष्टये ।। ईशावास्योपनिषत् : १५

Meaning

> Like a lid to a vessel, O sun your golden orb covers the entrance to the truth. Kindly open the entrance to lead me to the truth.

TIPS

1. Do it at sunrise and sunset, facing the Sun
2. Practice after loosening exercises before Asanas
3. Combination of Yogasana and Pranayama
4. Two modes of doing Surya Namaskar are 10 steps and 12 steps
5. With each round, chant BIJA MANTRA with the name of the SUN GOD

BIJA MANTRA: 12 STEPPED SALUTATION TO SUN

1. *Om Hram Mitraya Namah !*
   salutation to the friends of all
2. *Om Hrim Ravaye Namah !*
   salutation to one who shines
3. *Om Hrum Suryaya Namah !*
   salutation to one who induces activity
4. *Om Hraim Bhanave Namah !*
   salutation to one who illuminates
5. *Om Hroum Khagaya Namah !*
   salutation to one who moves quickly
6. *Om Hrah Pusne Namah !*
   salutation to one who gives strength
7. *Om hram Hiranyagarbhayaa Namah !*
   salutation to golden cosmic self
8. *Om Hrm Maricaye Namah !*
   salutation to lord of dawn
9. *Om Hrum Adityaya Namah !*
   salutation to son of aditi
10. *Om Hraim Savitre Namah !*
    salutation to stimulating power
11. *Om Hroum Arkaya Namah !*
    salutation to one who is fit to be praised
12. *Om Hrah Bhaskaraya Namah !*
    salutation to one who leads to enlightenment

Sun Salutation

Sthiti: Tadasana

Practice

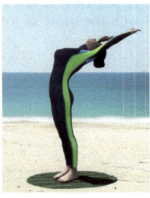

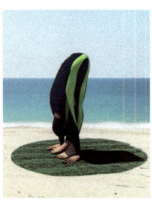

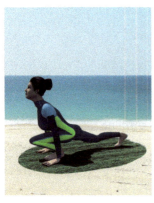

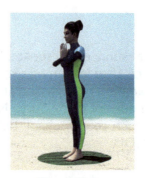

Pranayama

Stand erect with legs together. Bring the palms together to Namaska Mudra.

Step 1: Hastottanasana

1 - Inhale
Take the hands above the head while inhaling and bend the trunk backwards.

Step 2: Padahastasana

2 - Exhale
Bend the body forward while exhaling.
Touch the forehead to the knees.
Keep the palms on the floor on either side of the feet.

Step 3: Asvasancalanasana

3 - Inhale
In this step breathe in and kick the right leg back.
Push the buttock forward and downward so that the left leg is perpendicular to the ground.
Look up.

Practice

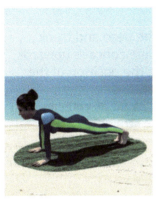

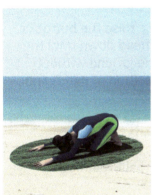

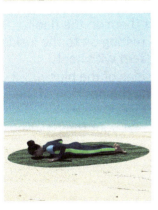

Step 4: Chaturanga Dandasana

4 – Exhale

In this step, exhale and take the left leg also back, resting only on the palms and toes.
Keep the body straight from head to toes inclined to the ground at about 30O. Keep the neck in line with the back.

Step 5: Sasankasana

5 – Exhale & Normal Breathing

While inhaling, bend the legs at the knees and rest them on the floor with buttocks resting on the inside surface of the feet with heels touching the sides of the hips without altering the position of the palms and toes. Exhale as you rest your forehead on the floor. Then relax in normal breathing.

Step 6: Astanga Namaskara

6 – Exhale & Bahya Kumbhaka

While exhaling without shifting the positions of hands and toes, glide the body forward and hold your breath (Bahya Kumbhaka) and rest the forehead, chest, hands, knees, and toes on the ground. Raise the buttock off the ground.
Note that eight points of the body are in contact with the ground – hence the name Astanga Namaskara (Salutation with eight parts).

Practice

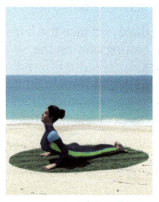

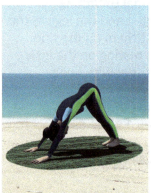

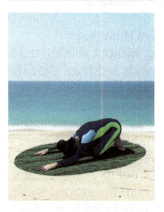

Step 7: Bhujangasana

7 - Inhale
Inhale; raise the head and trunk making the spine concave upwards without lifting the position of the hands and feet.
Arch the back as far as you can until the elbows are straight.
Keep the knees off the ground.

Step 8: Parvatasana

8 - Exhale
While exhaling, raise the buttocks, and push the head down until the heels touch the ground without shifting the position of hands and feet.

Step 9: Sasankasana

9 – Exhale & Normal Breathing
Same as step 5.
While inhaling, bend the legs at the knees and rest them on the floor with buttocks resting on to the inside surface of the feet with heels touching the sides of the hips without altering the position of the palms and toes.
Exhale as you rest your forehead on the floor. Then relax in normal breathing.

Practice

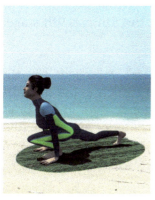

Step 10: Asvasancalanasana

10 - Inhale

Inhale and bring the right leg in between the two hands. Arch the back concave upwards as in step 3 until the right leg is perpendicular to the ground.

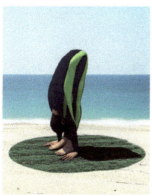

Step 11: Padahastasana

11- Exhale

Exhale and bring the left foot forward next to the right foot and reach down with your upper body to touch the forehead to the knees as in step 2.

Step 12: Hastottanasana

12 – Inhale

Take the hands above the head while inhaling and bend the trunk backward.
While exhaling, come to Pranamasana and then come back to Sthiti.

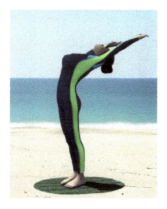

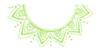

This completes one round of Surya Namaskar Repeat 3 rounds and reach up to 12 rounds in one month

Note: in the 10-steps of - Surya Namaskar the 5th and 9th stages are omitted.

The prolonged pronunciation of 'Omkar' followed by the Bijaksara, 'Ha' and the sounds 'R' and 'M' which come in every Mantra influences and stimulates the nerve centers in the brain corresponding to the respiratory, circulatory and digestive systems, making them more active, efficient and healthy.

Benefits:

1. Increases flexibility of the body.
2. Tones muscles.
3. Improves circulation.
4. Harmonies breathing.
5. Releases Prana blocks.
6. Prepares for Asanas and Pranayama.

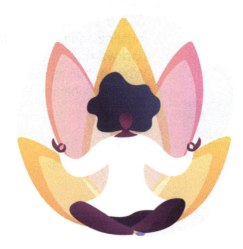

4: Yog Asanas

KICK OFF

"Asanas are physical postures designed to enhance both physical health and mental well-being. The term originates from Sanskrit, meaning 'posture' or 'pose.' Asanas extend beyond the boundaries of the physical realm, offering spiritual contentment. They serve to improve body posture and expand the chest while stretching the spine."

Any system or process is accepted by youngsters if it can prove its usefulness in their day-to-day life. Now society is all set for Yoga. Studies prove that asanas can help to lose weight, stabilize period cramps, and shoot up the health of the heart and digestion. Asanas can even be performed anywhere, in an open place, at home without any instruments. Asanas essentially work to lubricate the muscles, joints, ligaments and other parts of the body. This helps to increase circulation and flexibility. They also help better the internal body health as different asanas work on different internal parts of the body. So, if you have any health issue, you can look for a relevant asana to practice to take care of the ailment. Sometimes, people feel lethargic and drained without having any underlying medical condition. Practicing daily asanas can boost energy and also improve health. If incorporated into your daily busy schedule, asanas can help to retain the mind-body balance.

Yoga asanas are performed in

1. **Standing**
2. **Sitting**
3. **Prone**
4. **Supine**

Yoga asana keeps the whole body in proper condition. Regular practice of asanas is useful to reduce fat in various parts of our bodies. This will help to reduce weight and maintain the body in proper health in the long run.

I - Standing Postures

A: Ardha Kati Chakrasana (Half-wheel posture)

Sthiti: Tadasana

Practice

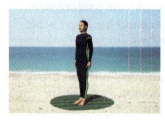

1. While inhaling, slowly raise the right arm sideways up

2. At the horizontal level turn the palm upwards

3. Continue to raise the arm with deep inhaling vertically until the biceps touch the right ear

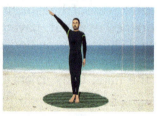

4. Stretch the right arm upwards

5. While exhaling, bend the trunk slowly to the left

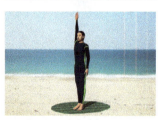

6. The left palm slides down along the left thigh as far as possible

7. Do not bend the right elbow or the knees

8. Maintain for about a minute with normal breathing

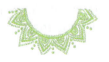

9. Slowly while coming back to the vertical position inhale and stretch the right arm up, feel the pull along a straight line from the waist up to the fingers

10. Bring the right arm down as you exhale to the Sthiti position

11. Come back to Tadasana Sthiti

12. Repeat the same on the other side

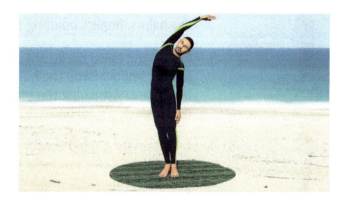

Repeat the same on the other side,

Benefits
1. Reduces fat in the waist region
2. Stimulates sides of the body
3. Gives lateral bending to the spine
4. Improves liver function

No Limitation - Any one can do.

Key Points
1. Elbows straight
2. Knees straight
3. Lateral bend only at the waist
4. Left arm hanging freely

"Healthy habits in childhood plant seeds of well-being that grow into a lifetime of good health."

B: Ardha Chakrasana (Half-wheel posture)

Sthiti: Tadasana

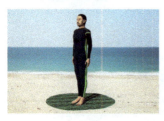
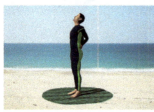

Practice

1. Sthiti Tadasana
2. Support the back at the waist with the palms, fingers pointing forwards
3. Inhale and bend backwards from the lumbar region. Drop the head backward, stretching the muscles of the neck
4. Maintain for a minute with normal breathing
5. Return to Sthiti
6. Relax in Tadasana

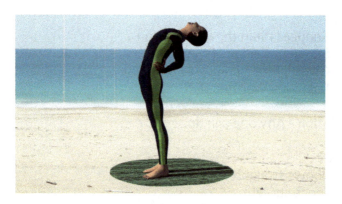

Benefits
1. Makes the spine flexible
2. Stimulates the spinal nerves
3. Circulation of blood into the head
4. Expands chest and shoulders

Limitations
1. Cardiac Problems
2. Recent abdominal surgery
3. Vertigo

Key Points
1. All the fingers pointed forward
2. Wrist as close as possible
3. Elbows are as close as possible
4. Knees straight
5. Head hanging freely with relaxed neck muscles
6. Bend from the waist

Attractions & Distractions

In our day-to-day lives, we're constantly surrounded by attractions and distractions. Friends, the allure of social media, and tempting foods often pull us away from our intended path. Yet, despite these influences, it's crucial to stand resolute in our commitment to two fundamental pillars: maintaining a healthy diet and embracing yoga. These choices are pivotal for our holistic development across five distinct levels.In the face of the distractions that seek to derail our wellness journey, let us remember the profound impact that a healthy diet and yoga can have on our lives. By remaining steadfast, we not only fortify our bodies but also empower our minds, emotions, and spirits. Let's make a conscious choice to rise above the allure of momentary pleasures and commit to our long-term well-being. In doing so, we will experience growth and transformation across these five interconnected dimensions of our being.

C: Padahastasana (Forward-Bend Posture)
Sthiti: Tadasana

Practice

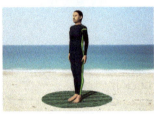
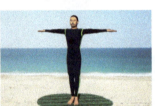
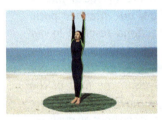
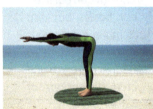

1. Stand erect with legs together

2. Inhale slowly and raise the arms sideways

3. At this horizontal level, turn the palms upwards

4. Continue to inhale and move the arms upwards until the biceps touch the ears. Turn the palms forward

5. Stretch up the body from the waist

6. Keeping the lower back concave, exhale and bend forward until the trunk is parallel to the ground. Stretch out the shoulders at the horizontal plane and inhale

7. Exhale while going down further until the entire palm rests on the ground and the chin touches the knees

8. Maintain this final posture for about 2-3 minutes without bending the knees

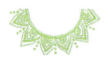

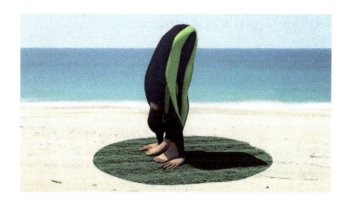

Benefits
1. Makes the spine flexible
2. Strengthens the thighs
3. Helps to prevent constipation
4. Helps in menstrual disorders
5. Improves digestion
6. Enhances blood flow to the head region

Limitation
1. Vertigo
2. Hypertension
3. Cervical Spondylosis
4. Cardiac Problems
5. Spinal Problems

Key Points
1. Don't bend the knees
2. Bend from lower back
3. Maintain the arms in such a way that the biceps are in contact with the ear lobes
4. Don't overstrain

"In the fight against childhood obesity, every small step towards healthier living makes a significant impact."

D: Trikonasana (Triangle Posture)

Sthiti: Tadasana

Practice

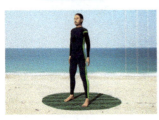

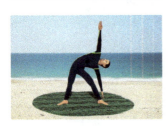

1. While inhaling, spread the feet apart by about a meter and raise both hands slowly till they reach the horizontal position simultaneously

2. Slowly bend to the right side until the right-hand reaches the right foot. The left arm is straight up, in line with the right hand. Palms face forward. Stretch up the left arm and see along the fingers

3. Maintain for about one minute with normal breathing

4. Return slowly to Sthiti

5. Repeat on the left side

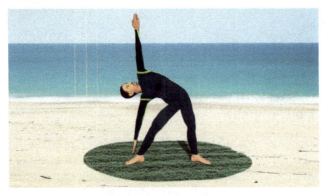

Benefits
1. Helps in preventing flat feet
2. Strengthens the calf and thigh muscles
3. Strengthens the waist muscles
4. Make the spine flexible

Limitation
1. Undergone recent abdominal surgery
2. Cardiac Problems
3. Slip disc
4. Sciatica

Key Points
1. Lateral bend only from the waist
2. Legs parallel to each other
3. Left palm facing forward in the final position
4. Hands at 180

Well-being

We need to shift our mindset and embrace a holistic approach to health. This means acknowledging that obesity is a complex issue that requires multifaceted solutions. It's about making gradual changes in our lifestyle, finding ways to incorporate yoga into our daily routines, and recognizing the importance of pranayama & meditation for mental and emotional well-being. Let's stop fixating on shortcuts and excuses. Let's acknowledge that our health is worth investing time and effort into. It's time to break free from the limitations we've imposed on ourselves and explore the various avenues available for improving our well-being. It's time to empower ourselves with ancient knowledge of yoga, and take proactive steps toward a healthier life.

E: Parivrtta Trikonasana (Crossed Triangle Posture)

Sthiti: Tadasana

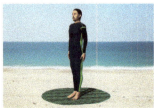

1. While inhaling, spread the legs apart by about a meter by moving the right leg away from the left

2. While exhaling, the right hand is taken down to the ground on the outside of the left foot, while the left arm is raised up to the vertical position

3. Turn the face up to look at the raised hand

4. Maintain the final posture for one minute with normal breathing

5. Return to Sthiti and repeat the same to the left side

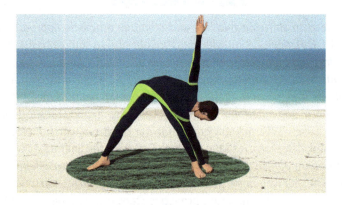

Benefits
1. Gives rotational movement to the spine
2. Strengthens the thigh muscles

Limitations
1. Spinal problems
2. Heart problems
3. Hypertension

Key Points
1. Bend from lower back
2. Knees straight
3. Hands in 180 degrees
4. Foot parallel to each other

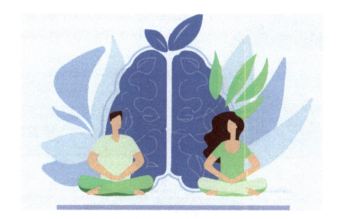

II - Sitting Postures

A: Vajrasana (The Ankle Posture)

Sthiti: Dandasana

Practice

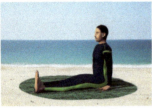

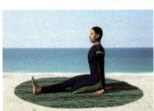

1. Fold the right leg & bring the right heel under the right buttock

2. Sitting on the right heel, fold the left leg and bring the left heel under the left buttock

3. Sit erect comfortably with the buttocks resting both the heels and palms resting on the thighs

4. In the final posture, the soles of the feet face upwards, heels are kept together and the entire weight of the body is felt on the back of the feet

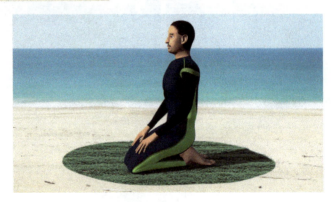

Limitations: Rheumatic Problems

Key Points
1. Heels together
2. Weight of the body on the back of the feet

Benefits
1. Keeps the spine erect and removes drowsiness
2. Activates Vajranadi
3. Increases awareness
4. Reduces Varicose veins

Reduce

B: Ustrasana (Camel Posture)

Sthiti: Dandasana

Practice

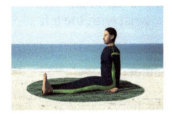

1. Sit in Vajrasana
2. Stand on the knees
3. Place the palms on the waist with fingers pointing forwards
4. Inhale and bend the trunk backwards and place the palms on the heels

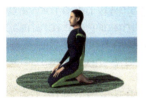 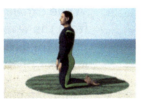 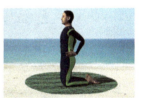

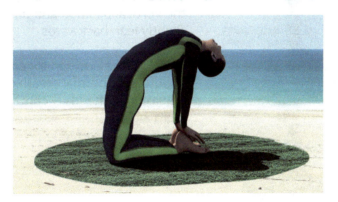

Benefits
1. Push the abdomen forward and see that the thighs are perpendicular to the ground
2. Both legs may be separated by shoulder width apart initially; with practice one can bring them together

C : Sasankasana (Moon Posture)

Sthiti: Dandasana

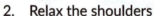

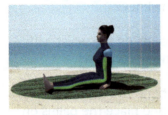

1. Take the hands behind the back, make a fist of the right hand and hold the right wrist with the left hand

2. Relax the shoulders

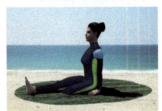

3. While inhaling, bend backwards from the waist opening up the chest

4. While exhaling slowly bend forward from the waist bringing the forehead on to the ground in front of the knees. Collapse the shoulders

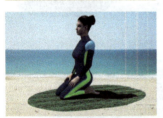

5. While inhaling slowly come up to the vertical position and then slightly lean backwards

6. Maintain the position for one minute with normal breathing Release your hands & come back to sthiti

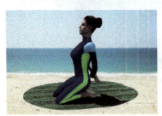

"A healthy child is a happy child; let's build a future where obesity is replaced with joy and vitality."

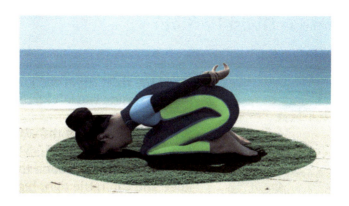

Benefits
1. Enhances blood flow to the head
2. Stimulates the brain
3. Flexibility to the spine, knees, and ankles
4. Good for breathing ailments

Limitations: Gastritis and Peptic Ulcer

Key Points
1. While bending forward allow the abdomen to touch the thighs, chest to knees, and forehead to the ground
2. Hips in contact with heels in the final position
3. Shoulders are loose, free and relaxed
4. While coming up first the head raises up then the chest then the abdomen

"Obesity doesn't run in families, it's the lifestyle that runs in families."

D: Vakrasana (Twist Posture)

Sthiti: Dandasana

Practice

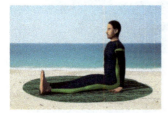

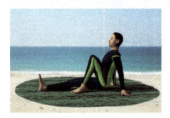

1. Bend the right leg at the knee and place it beside the left knee

2. Straighten and twist the waist towards the right as you exhale. Bring the left arm around the right knee and catch the right big toe

3. Take the right arm back and keep the palm on the ground in such a way that the trunk is kept erect with a proper twist

4. After maintaining for about a minute with normal breathing return to Sthiti and relax for a while in SithilaDandasana

5. Repeat the same on the other side

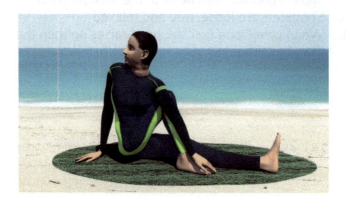

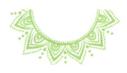

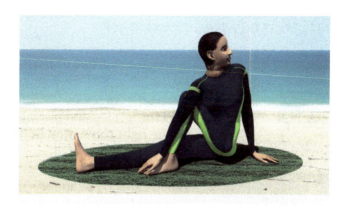

Benefits
1. Flexibility to the spine
2. Tones up the spinal nerves
3. Cures constipation
4. Improves lung capacity

Limitations: Gastritis and Peptic Ulcer

Key Points
1. Middle of the foot by the side of the knee
2. The pressure of raised leg on the abdomen
3. The forward stretched leg should be maintained straight

"Childhood obesity is a silent epidemic that can only be defeated with awareness, education, and action."

E: Spinal Stretch (with folded legs)

Sthiti: Dandasana

Practice

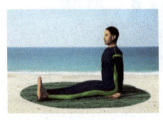

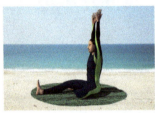

1. Fold the left leg and place the heel on the right thigh, stretch up your hands above the head

2. While exhaling bend forward, hold your right toe with the hands, and try to touch the forehead to the right knee

3. While inhaling, come up with your hands stretched up. Do this for 10 times

4. Repeat the same on the other side for 10 times

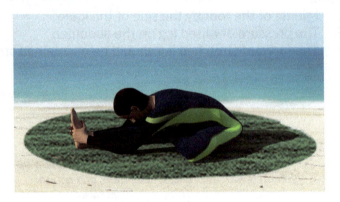

Notes
1. While bending forward do not bend the knee
2. Gradually increase the speed

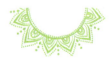

F: Bhunamanasana Stretch (spinal twist prostration pose)

Sthiti: Dandasana

Practice

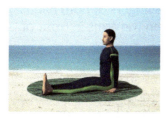

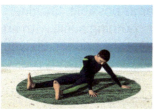

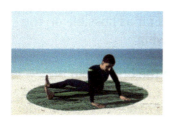

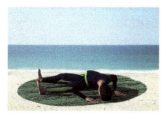

1. Sit with the spine erect and the legs outstretched
2. Place the hands to the side of the right hip
3. Move the right hand back slightly further behind the body with the fingers pointing backward
4. Twist the trunk 90 degrees to the right, using the arms and shoulders in level
5. Slowly bend the torso and bring the forehead to the floor
6. If possible keep both buttocks on the floor
7. Hold the final position for a short time
8. Slowly raise and return to the sthiti
9. Repeat the movement on the other side. This completes one round
10. Practice up to 5 rounds

Notes
1. Breathing: Inhale while facing forward
2. Retain the breath in while twisting
3. Exhale while bending
4. Retain the breath out in the final position
5. Inhale while raising the trunk
6. Exhale while re-centering the body

G: Chakki Chalana Stretch

Sthiti: Dandasana

Practice

Stage 1:

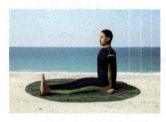

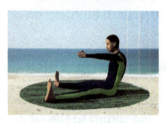

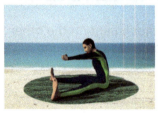

1. Separate the legs by about one foot. Interlock the fingers of both hands and straighten the arms in front of the chest

2. Keep the arms straight and horizontal throughout the practice; do not bend the elbows. Bend forward as far as possible. Imagine the action of churning a mill with an old-fashioned stone grinder. Swivel to the right so that the hands pass above the right toes and as far to the right as possible

3. Lean back as far as possible on the backward swing

4. Try to move the body from the waist. On the forward swing, bring the arms and hands to the left side, over the left toes and then back to the center position

5. One rotation is one round

6. Practice 5 to 10 rounds clockwise and then the same number of rounds anti-clockwise

> *The rise of childhood obesity has placed the health of an entire generation at risk.*
> *- Tom Vilsack*

Stage 2:

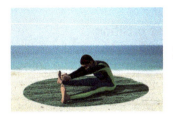

1. In the same sitting position, separate the legs as wide as possible, keeping them straight

2. Make large, circular movements over both feet, again trying to take the hands over the toes on the forward swing and coming as far back as possible on the backward swing

3. Practice 10 times in each direction

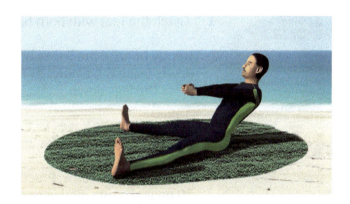

Note
1. Breathing: Inhale while leaning back. Exhale while moving forward

The people in power have created an obesity epidemic.
- Robert Atkins

Reduce

H: Full Butterfly

Sthiti: Dandasana

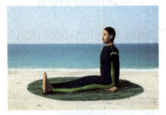

Practice

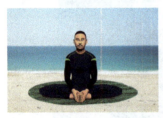

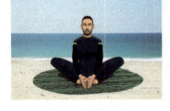

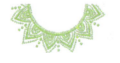

Stage 1:
1. Sit in the base position
2. Bend the knees and bring the soles of the feet together, keeping the heels as close to the body as possible
3. Fully relax the inner thigh muscles

Stage 2:
1. Catch the feet with both hands
2. Gently bounce the knees up and down, using the elbows as levers to press the legs down
3. Try to touch the knees to the ground on the downward stroke
4. Do not use any force. Practice 30 to 50 up and down movements
5. Keep the soles of the feet together. Place the hands on the knees
6. Using the palms, gently push the knees down towards the floor, allowing them to spring up again
7. Do not force this movement. Repeat 20 to 30 times
8. Straighten the legs and relax

Note
1. Breathing: Normal breathing, unrelated to the practice

III - Prone

A: Bhujangasana (Serpent Posture)

Sthiti: Prone Posture

Practice

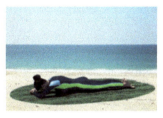

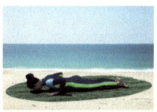

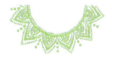

1. Bend the arms at the elbows and place the palms beside the lower chest at the level of the last rib exerting the least pressure on the palms

2. Keep the elbows close to each other and let them not spread out

3. Inhale and come up

4. Arch the dorsal spine and neck backwards as far as you can

5. Keep the body below the navel in touch with the ground

6. Maintain the final position with normal breathing for one minute with the least pressure on the palms

7. While exhaling, come back to the Sthiti position

8. Relax in Makarāsana

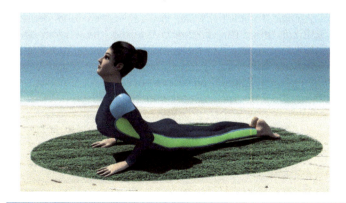

Benefits
1. Flexibility to the dorsal spine
2. Strengthens the spinal muscles
3. Prevents back pain
4. Reduces abdominal fat
5. Useful in managing bronchial problems

Limitations
1. Recent abdominal surgery
2. Cervical spondylosis

Key Points
1. Palms by the sides of the last rib bones
2. Elbows as close to the body as possible
3. The body should be raised up to that the extent the navel is about to leave the ground
4. Legs and feet together and on the ground

Pancha Kosha

Childhood obesity, a pressing modern health concern, can be analyzed through the lens of the Pancha Kosha, a concept from ancient yogic philosophy that describes the five sheaths or layers of existence. In this context, childhood obesity is not just a physical issue but can also affect the annamaya kosha (the physical body) by creating imbalances and health complications. Furthermore, it can influence the pranamaya kosha (the vital energy body) by disrupting the flow of life force energy due to excess weight. Obesity can also have an impact on the manomaya kosha (the mental body) as it may lead to psychological challenges like low self-esteem and depression. Finally, it can affect the vijnanamaya kosha (the wisdom body) by hindering one's capacity to make informed choices about nutrition and lifestyle. Therefore, addressing childhood obesity involves considering its implications on all levels of existence, emphasizing not only physical health but also mental, emotional, and spiritual well-being.

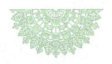

B: Parvatasana (Mountain Pose)

Sthiti: Prone Posture

Practice

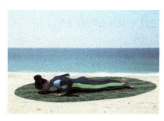
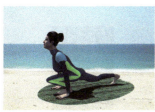

1. Take the left foot back beside the right foot

2. Simultaneously, raise the buttocks and lower the head between the arms, so that the back and legs form two sides of a triangle

3. The legs and arms should be straight in the final position

4. Try to keep the heels on the floor in the final pose and bring the head towards the knees

5. Do not strain

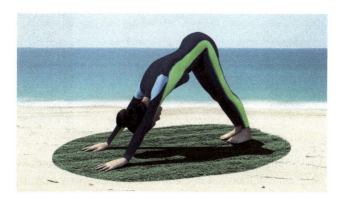

Benefits
1. This pose strengthens the nerves and muscles in the arms and legs
2. The spinal nerves are toned and circulation is stimulated especially in the upper spine, between the shoulder blades
3. It gives a natural massage to the heart and lung muscles
4. It is very useful in relieving lumber, spinal, shoulder, knee and ankle pains and varicose veins

Reduce

Note
1. Breathing: Exhale while taking the left leg back

Limitations
1. Those who have recently undergone abdominal, and knee joint surgery avoid this posture
2. Parvatāsana should not be practiced with problems of shoulder dislocation
3. Those having complaints of a reeling sensation should not practice it

---

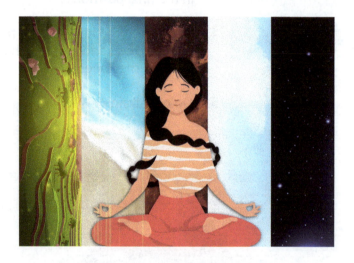

Childhood obesity, a growing concern in today's world, finds insights and potential solutions in ancient sciences. Drawing from age-old wisdom, these sciences emphasize the harmony between the body, mind, and spirit. They recognize that a balanced lifestyle, including dietary habits and physical activity, is essential for holistic well-being. The principles of moderation, mindful eating, and regular exercise, as advocated by ancient sciences, can play a pivotal role in addressing the complex issue of child obesity. By incorporating these timeless practices into modern life, we have the opportunity to nurture healthier, happier, and more resilient generations.

C: Dhanurasana (Bow Posture)

Sthiti: Prone Posture

Practice

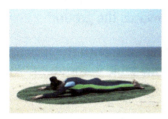

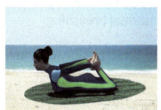

1. Bend the knees and hold the ankles by the palms

2. As you inhale, raise the head and the chest upwards. Pull the legs outwards and backwards so that the spine is arched back like a bow

3. Stabilize (rest) on the abdomen

4. Do not bend the elbows. Look up & Keep the toes together

6. Maintain for about half a minute with normal breathing

7. Slowly come back to Sthiti while exhaling. Relax in Makarāsana

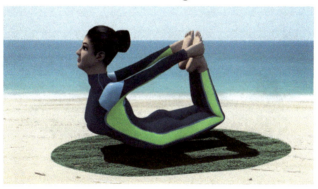

Limitations: Any health problem

Key Points
1. Both feet together   2. Hold only the ankles, not the toes
3. Give a backward push to the legs

Benefits
1. Stimulates and slims the body
2. Gives good stimulation and flexibility to the back

D: Salabhasana Both Legs (Locust Posture)

Sthiti: Prone Posture

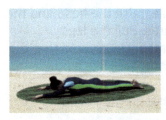

1. Make fists of your palms with the thumbs tucked in and place them under the thighs, with the back of the hands towards the ground

2. While inhaling raise both the legs up as far as comfortable without bending the knees

3. Maintain this position for about one minute with normal breathing

4. Come back to Sthiti position while exhaling

5. Relax in Makarāsana

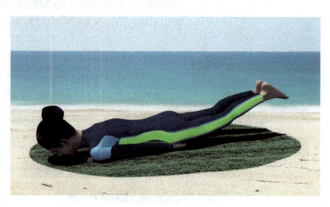

Limitations: Cardiac patients.

Key Points
1. Both feet together
2. Do not bend knees
3. Chin on the ground
4. Awareness of the thyroid
5. Give a backward push to the feet to raise up

Benefits
1. Helps to manage sciatica and lower backache
2. Tones the hip muscles

IV - Supine

A: Chakra Padasana (Leg Rotation)

Sthiti: Supine Posture

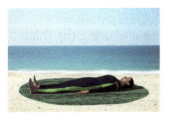

1. Lie in the base position
2. Raise the right leg 5 cm from the ground, keeping the knee straight
3. Rotate the entire leg clockwise 10 times in as large a circle as possible
4. The heel should not touch the floor at any time during the rotation
5. Rotate 10 times in the opposite direction
6. Repeat with the left leg
7. Do not strain
8. Rest in the base position introducing abdominal breathing until the respiration returns to normal

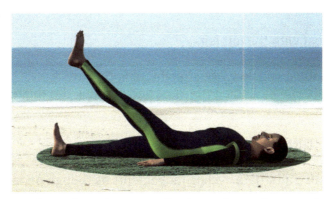

Note: Breathing: Breathe normally throughout the practice

Benefits
1. Good for hip joints, obesity, and toning of abdominal and spinal muscles

B: Pada Sanchalana (Cycling)

Sthiti: Supine Posture

Practice

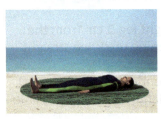

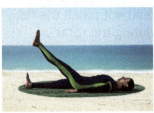

Stage 1:

1. Lie in the base position
2. Raise the right leg
3. Bend the knee and bring the thigh to the chest
4. Raise and straighten the leg completely. Then, lower the straight leg in a forward movement
5. Bend the knee and bring it back to the chest to complete the cycling movement
6. The heel should not touch the floor during the movement
7. Repeat 10 times in a forward direction and then 10 times in reverse
8. Repeat with the left leg
9. Breathing: Inhale while straightening the leg. Exhale while bending the knee and bringing the thigh to the chest

Stage 2: Raise both legs

1. Practice alternate cycling movements as though pedaling a bicycle
2. Practice 10 times forward and then 10 times backward
3. Breathing: Breathe normally throughout

Stage 3: Raise both legs and keep them together throughout the practice
1. Bring the knees as close as possible to the chest on the backward

2. Movement and straighten the legs fully on the forward movement. Slowly lower the legs together, keeping the knees straight, until the legs are just above the floor. Then bend the knees and bring them back to the chest. Practice 3 to 5 forward cycling movements and the same in reverse.

3. Do not strain

4. Breathing: Inhale while straightening the legs. Exhale while bending the legs to the chest

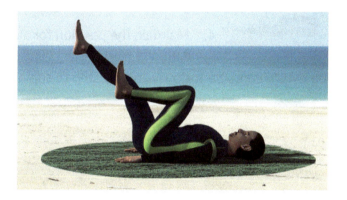

Benefits
1. Good for hip and knee joints. Strengthens abdominal and lower back muscles

Note
1. Keep the rest of the body, including the head, flat on the floor throughout the practice
2. After completing each stage remain in the base position and relax until the respiration returns to normal
3. If cramping is experienced in the abdominal muscles inhale deeply, gently pushing out the abdomen, and then relax the whole body with exhalation. Do not strain; this applies especially to stage 3

C: Chakrasana (Wheel Posture)

Sthiti: Supine Posture

Practice

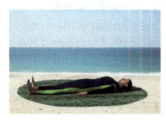

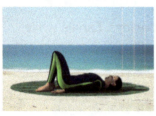

1. Take the hands up and place the palms on either side of the head on the ground under the shoulders with fingers pointing towards the back

2. Bend the knees and fold the legs, and place the heels on the outer side of the buttocks

3. With palms and the soles of the feet as four points of support, raise the trunk off the ground with an inhalation arching the entire body convex upwards to look like a wheel

4. Maintain the position for about half a minute with normal breathing

5. As you exhale come back slowly step by step to supine Sthiti

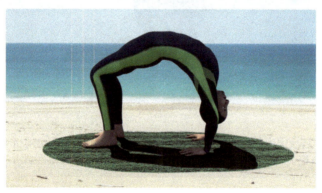

Limitations: Any kind of disease

Practice
1. Bring the heels closure to the buttocks
2. While coming back first head should reach the ground then the back and then the buttocks

Benefits
1. Brings flexibility to the spine & stimulates all parts of the body
3. Strengthens the arms, shoulders, and legs

D: Setu Bandhasana

Setu means bridge. Setu Bandha means the construction of bridges. In the posture, the whole body forms an arch, and is supported at one end by the crown of the head and the other ends on the feet, hence the name.

Sthiti: Supine Posture

Practice

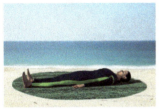
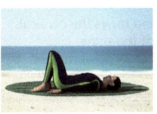
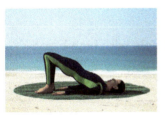

1. Lie flat on the back of the floor. Take a few deep breaths

2. Bend the knees, widen the legs at the knees, and bring the heels towards the buttocks

3. Keep the heels together and rest the outer sides firmly on the floor

4. Bring the hands by the side of the head and with an exhalation raise the trunk and arch the body up to rest the crown of the head on the floor. Pull the head far as back as possible by stretching the neck up and lifting the dorsal and lumbar region of the back off the floor

5. Fold the arms across the chest and hold the left elbow with the right hand and the right elbow with the left hand. Take 2 or 3 breaths

6. Exhale, draw the hips up, and stretch out the legs until they are straight. Join the feet and press them firmly to the ground. The whole body now forms a bridge or an arch. One end of it is supported by the crown of the head and the other end is on the feet

7. Hold this position for a few seconds with normal breathing

8. Exhale, unfold the arms and place the hands on the floor, bend the knees, lower the legs and trunk to the floor, release the head grip, straighten the neck, lie flat on the back and relax

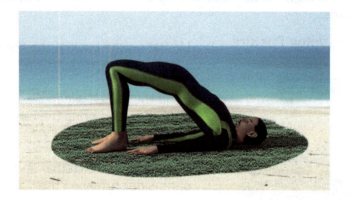

Benefits
1. The Asana strengthens the neck and tones the cervical, dorsal, lumbar and sacral regions of the spine
2. The extensor muscles of the back grow powerful and the hips are contracted and hardened
3. The pineal, pituitary, thyroid and adrenal glands are bathed in blood and function properly

Limitations
1. This Āsana is not practiced by people with high blood pressure, weak neck muscles and heart conditions.

> "Yog is not about touching your toes, it's about what you learn on the way down.
> - Jigar Gor

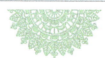

E: Naukasana

Sthiti: Supine Posture

Practice

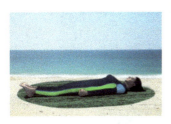
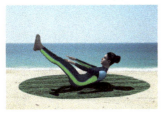

1. Lie in the base position, palms down

2. Keep your eyes open throughout

3. Breathe in deeply. Hold the your breath and then raise the legs, arms, shoulders, head, and trunk off the ground

4. The shoulders and feet should not be more than 15 cm off the floor. Balance the body on the buttocks and keep the spine straight

5. The arms should be hold at the same level and in line with the toes

6. The hands should be open with the palms down

7. Look towards the toes

8. Remain in the final position and hold your breath. Count 1 to 5 mentally or more if possible

9. Breathe out and return to the supine position. Be careful not to injure the back of the head while returning to the floor

10. Relax the whole body

11. This is one round. Practice 3 to 5 rounds

12. Relax in savāsana after each round, gently pushing out the abdomen with inhalation to relax the stomach muscles

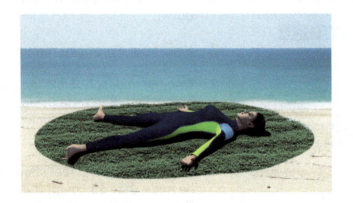

Limitations: People who have abdominal surgery should not do this Āsana

Notes
1. Breathing: Inhale before raising the body
2. Retain the breath while raising, tensing, and lowering the body
3. Exhale in the base position

Benefits
1. This Āsana stimulates the muscular, digestive, circulatory, nervous and hormonal systems, tones all the organs and removes lethargy
2. It is especially useful for eliminating nervous tension and bringing about deep relaxation

Continuous practice of yog gives deep relaxation at muscular level.

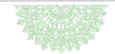

5: Breathing Techniques

KICK OFF

This practice is like saying 'hello' to your breath. A simple technique that introduces the practitioners to their own breathing patterns and respiratory system.

Awareness of the breathing process in itself is sufficient to slow down the respiratory rate and establish a more relaxed rhythm.

This in terms helps to center the thoughts, build focus and calm the mind. The respiratory system is a bridge between the conscious and subconscious, voluntary & involuntary, which means body & mind. The immune system must be strong to fight in any form of the disease, be it Covid or other seasonal fevers.

Breathing techniques help in strengthening all the internal parts of the body. The objective of breathing practises which are incorporated in our protocol, bringing into action all the lobes of the lungs for full utilization, to normalize the breathing rate and also make breathing uniform, continuous & rhythmic.

Breathing exercise is very helpful to de-stress.

> *Breathing Techniques helps to slow down breath and maintaining balance at Pranic level.*

A: Hands In And Out Breathing

Sthiti: Tadasana

Relax: Sithila Tadasana

Practice

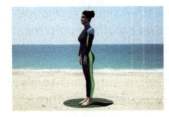

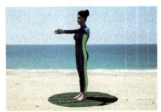

1. Stretch out your arms in front, in level with your shoulders and bring the palms together

2. Inhaling spread your arms sideways in a horizontal plane

3. While exhaling, bring the arms forward with palms touching each other

4. Repeat 5 times making your arms movements continuous and synchronizing with the breath flowing in and out rhythmically

5. Relax in Sithila Tadasana. Feel the changes in the breath and the body, especially the arms, shoulders and the back of the neck

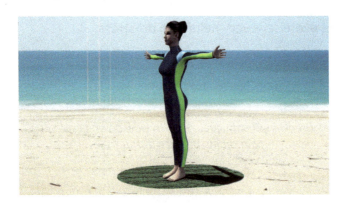

Feel the changes in: 1. Breath 2. Arms
3. Shoulders 4. Back 5. Neck

B: Hands Stretch Breathing

Sthiti: Tadasana

Relax: Sithila Tadasana

At 90, 135, and 180 degrees

Practice

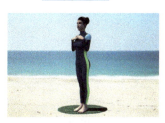

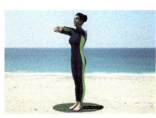

90 degree

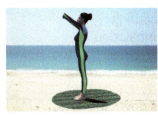

135 degree

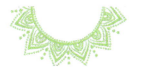

Stage 1:
1. While inhaling, stretch the arms straight out in front of your body so that the arms are at shoulders level

2. At the same time twist the hands so that the palms face outwards

3. Fully stretch the arms, but do not strain

4. While exhaling, reverse the process and bring the palms back on to the chest

5. Collapse the shoulders again

6. This is one round. Repeat 5 times

Stage 2:
1. Repeat the same movements now stretching the arms above the forehead at an angle of 135 Degree

2. Repeat 5 times

Stage 3: Vertical
1. Repeat the same movements, this time stretching the arms vertically above the head

2. Repeat 5 times

Reduce

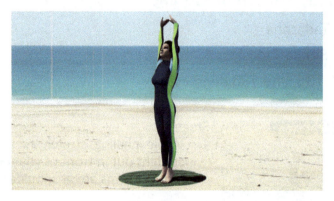

180 degree

Benefits
1. Helps in opening the lower, middle and the upper part of the chest
2. Balancing Prana
3. Promotes rhythmic breathing
4. Increases awareness of breathing
5. Improves concentration and calms down the mind

Note
1. Collapse the shoulders at the beginning and end of each cycle
2. Maintain perfect awareness of breathing
3. Exhalation should be longer than inhalation
4. If required, it can be practiced sitting in a chair too
5. Synchronize the breathing with hand movements
6. Balance the Prana in the chest
7. Improves concentration and calms down the mind

Yog practices helps to Increase creativity and will powers at mental level.

Reduce

C: Ankle Stretch Breathing

Sthiti: Tadasana

Relax: Sithila Tadasana

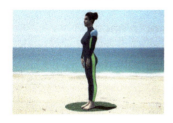

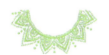

1. Eyes open
2. Fix your gaze on a point in front of you
3. While inhaling , raise your hands & stretch the Ankles
4. Feel the stretch from ankle to finger
5. As you exhale bring your hand & heels down
6. Relax in a standing position. Enjoy the stability
7. Repeat five to ten types

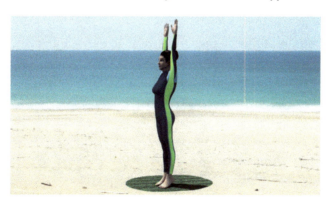

Benefits
1. Increases awareness of breathing
2. Strengthens the clavicular muscles
3. Improves awareness of the middle part of the lungs
4. Improves the capacity to focus
5. Relaxes and balances the body
6. Calms down the mind
7. Balances the Prana

D: Dog Breathing

Sthiti: Vajrasana

Relax: Sasankasana

Practice

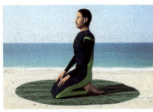

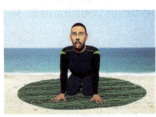

1. Place the palms of the hand on the ground beside the knees
2. Make the spine slightly concave & fix the gaze straight ahead
3. Keep your mouth open
4. The tongue is pushed out to its maximum
5. Practice rapidly
6. Forceful inhalation & exhalation
7. Abdominal breathing
8. Repeat the practice for 30 seconds. Relax in Vajrasana

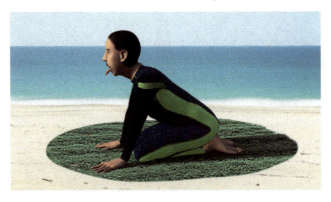

Limitations: 1. Epilepsy   2. High Blood Pressure

Benefits
1. Increased diaphragm contraction empties the lungs
2. Rapid exhalation cleanses the lungs
3. Increases awareness of the middle and lower part of the lungs
4. Open up Prana blocks
5. Calms down the mind

E: Rabbit Breathing

Sthiti: Vajrasana

Relax: Sasankasana

Practice

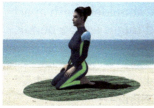
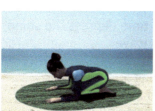
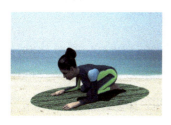
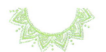

1. Keeping the knees together bend forward & rest the forearms on the floor, palms flat on the ground
2. Maintain the head at a distance of one hand length from the ground to the chin, and open your mouth partially. Produce the tongue partially. Touch the lower lip resting on the lower set of teeth
3. Gaze at a point two feet on the ground
4. Breathing rapidly through the mouth only using the upper part of the chest like a Rabbit. Continue for 20 to 40 stokes
5. Feel the air moving beautifully in and out of the lungs
6. Thoracic breathing
7. The abdomen is pressed on the thigh
8. No abdominal movement
9. Do not drop your head on the floor

Benefits
1. Helps in acute episodes of asthma
2. Develops voluntary control of muscles of lungs
3. Opens up Prana blocks
4. A quick way to calm down the mind

F: Tiger Breathing

Sthiti: Dandasana

Relax: Sasankasana

Practice

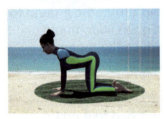

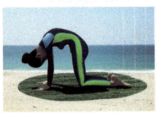

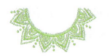

1. Come to Vajrasana
2. Lean forward and place the hands flat on the floor in line with the shoulders with fingers pointing forward. Arms, thighs & heels should be about one shoulder width apart. The arms and thighs are perpendicular to the floor
3. While in healing raise the head & look at the ceiling
4. At the same time depress the spine making it concave
5. While exhaling arch the spine upwards and bend the head downwards bringing the chin towards the chest
6. This constitutes one round of tiger breathing
7. Repeat 5 rounds

Notes
1. Ensure that you are comfortable with the posture before starting
2. Co-ordinate the movements with breathing
3. Eyes closed, practice with awareness
4. No movement of arms and thighs
5. Awareness of spinal movement

Benefits
1. Awareness and mastery over all three sections of the chest
2. Empties the lungs fully
3. Harmonize the muscles of respiration
4. Calm down the mind
5. Feedback of airway status by sound in case of asthmatics

G: Straight Leg Breathing

Sthiti: Supine Posture

Practice

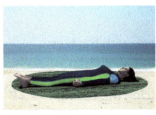
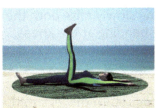

1. While inhaling slowly raise the right leg without bending the knee, as far as comfortable (up to 90°, if possible)

2. While exhaling return the leg to the floor as slowly as possible

3. Repeat the Practice with the left leg

4. This is one round. Perform 10 times

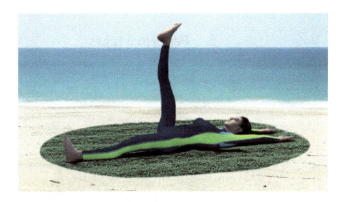

Notes
1. If you need, you can keep the arms by the side of your body with the palms facing the floor at any convenient position or at shoulder level
2. Do not bend the knee throughout the Practice
3. Do not disturb the leg lying straight on the ground in order to be able to raise the other leg further
4. Even if you can, do not raise the leg beyond 90°
5. Perfectly synchronize the breathing with leg movements
6. Maintain perfect breath awareness during the Practice

H: Both Legs Raising Breathing

Sthiti: Supine Posture

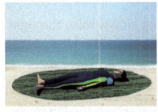

1. As you get stronger, you can do the leg-raising exercise with both legs. Avoid this exercise if you have low back pain

2. Lie on the back with the legs together, hands stretched out over the head, biceps touching the ears, and palms facing the ceiling

3. While inhaling slowly raise both the legs without bending at the knees, as far as comfortable (up to 90°, if possible)

4. While exhaling return the legs to the floor as slowly as possible

5. Perform 5 times

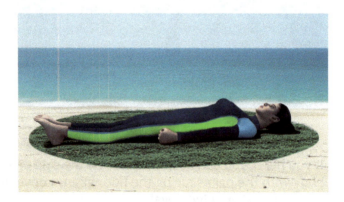

Notes
1. In the case of both legs, as you exhale and bring down the legs, there will be a tendency to fall down both legs too rapidly as they come close to the floor. So use strength and have control over the movement

I: Side Leg Raising

Sthiti: Supine Posture

Practice

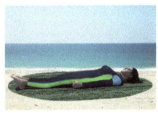

1. Lie down on the left side, with the head resting on the folded left arm
2. Support the back of the neck with the left hand
3. Place the right hand on the right thigh or in front of your chest
4. Keep the whole body as straight as possible
5. While inhaling slowly raise the right leg without bending the knee. Raise the leg as high as possible. Simultaneously stretch out the toes
6. While exhaling, slowly lower the right leg

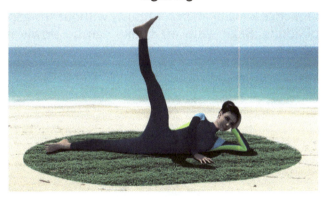

This is one round. Repeat this 5 times.
Repeat the same practice 5 times with the left leg while lying on the right side of the body.

Notes
1. While raising the leg you can maintain the balance, by pressing the palm on the ground
2. Feel the strong stimulation of the lateral stretch at the lumbar region

Reduce

6: Kapalbhati Preparatory practice for Pranayama

Kapalbhati is a rapid breathing technique that utilizes abdominal muscles for forceful active exhalation followed by slow, passive inhalation.

Since Kapalbhati removes toxins from the body, yoga experts call it 'shat kriya', which means the cleansing technique. Kapalbhati has to be practiced in a very steady posture, Padmasana, Siddhasana or Vajrasana with hands resting on the knees. These asanas are most suited to maintain posture during rapid breathing motion.

In normal breathing, inhalation is the active process while exhalation is passive. In Kapalbhati this is reversed. The abdominal muscles and the diaphragm are used forcefully to exhale the air. The abdominal muscles forcefully move inwards towards the diaphragm thereby throwing the air out.

The inhalation is done in a passive relaxed way to fill the lungs with fresh air. Practice kapalbhati in continusly without any gap between two respirations. Begin with 60 stroke can be slowly increse to 500 stokes.

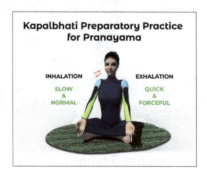

> Yog helps sharpening the intellect and calming down the mind at intellectual level.

Pranayama Techniques

KICK START

Pranayama is a profound practice that teaches the art of rhythmic, uniform, slow, and harmonious breathing. It extends beyond the mere act of breathing, for through mastery of the breath, one gains the ability to regulate and harmonize the body's functions. Pranayama acts as a bridge, forging a profound connection between the physical body, the mind, and the soul. By learning to control the breath, individuals unlock the potential to influence their entire being, fostering a deeper understanding of the intricate relationship between these facets of existence.

According to research, pranayama can promote relaxation and mindfulness. It's also proven that pranayama techniques support multiple aspects of physical health, including lung function, blood pressure, and brain function. Pranayama strengthens the muscles used in breathing, increasing our lung capacity and improving circulation throughout the body. By exhaling excess carbon dioxide and inhaling oxygen, breath-work can enhance the functioning of internal organs and boost the immune system.

Pranayama keeps vital energy in a proper condition. Daily pranayama trains the lungs and improves the capacity of the respiratory system immensely. Pranayama directly works on the nervous system. Pranayama positively affects the autonomic nervous system which controls and governs essential functions of the body like the heart rate, respiration and blood pressure. Regular practice of pranayama is useful to reduce fats in various parts of the body. This will help to reduce weight and maintain the body in proper health in the long run.

> *Yog enhances the happiness in life and equipoise at emotional level.*

7: Pranayama

A: Bhastrika Pranayama

The term Bhastrika means 'bellows'. We use the chest as bellows to have forceful inhalations and exhalations.

Sthiti: Sukhansana

Practice

1. Sit in Sukhansana or Padmasana with a spine erect

2. Relax the whole body and face with a smile

3. Inhale and exhale by expanding and compressing the chest vigorously like bellows. The speed of breathing should reach 120 strokes per minute when learned fully. In the beginning, it could be slower. But concentrate on full inhalations and exhalations

4. Stop after ten strokes to twenty as per capacity

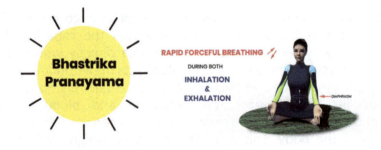

The breath stops automatically. Let it remain suspended as long as possible.

Do not exert. Enjoy the cessation of breath and thereby let the breath stop longer and longer.

Benefits
1. Relieves inflammation of the throat
2. Removes diseases of the nose and chest and eradicates Asthma etc
3. It breaks & dissolves the tumors
4. It is very much useful in Muscular Dystrophy and oxygen deficiency disorders
5. It brings about a proper balance of the tridosha. Vata, pitta, kapha & maintains their balance. Blood is purified and the body gets rid of foreign objects and toxins
6. Stabilises Prāṇa and calm the mind, & helps in the upward journey
7. Great freshness and agility are experienced in Bhastrika. It is not only the shattering of Tamas and stagnation but also the reduction of overtone and hypersensitivities to increase the functional efficiency of the cells
8. Helps to throw out toxins and cures illnesses of the respiratory tract

Limitations
1. This Pranayama should not be practiced by women who are pregnant
2. This Pranayama should not be practiced by people who have high blood pressure

Note
Bhastrika should be practiced with an empty stomach by normal healthy persons.

Pranayama practices manifest the innate divinity in man in all aspects of life.

B: Nadi Suddhi Pranayama

Sthiti: Vajrasana

Practice

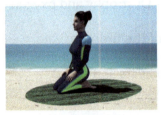
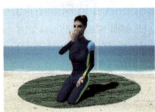
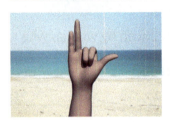

1. Sit in any meditative posture
2. Adopt Nasika Mudra
3. Close the right nostril with the right thumb and exhale completely through the left nostril. Then inhale deeply through the same left nostril
4. Close the left nostril with your ring and little finger of the Nasika Mudra, and release the right nostril. Now exhale slowly and completely through the right nostril
5. Inhale deeply through the same right nostril. Then close the right nostril and exhale through the left nostril. This is one round of Nadi Suddhi Pranayama
6. Repeat nine rounds

Note

1. This practice helps to maintain the balance between Nadis
2. If you feel headache, heaviness of the head, giddiness, uneasiness, etc. while doing this practice it means you are exerting much pressure on the lungs
3. The first symptoms of correct practice are the feeling of freshness, energy and lightness of the body and mind

Limitations: No Limitations.

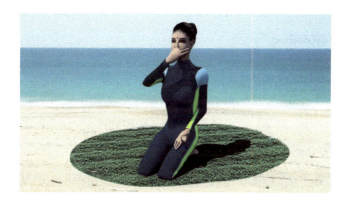

Benefits

Physical
It promotes balance between the two nostrils apart from cleansing the nasal tract. It increases vitality. The metabolic rate decreases as in the case of all other Pranayama practices. It increases the digestive fire and appetite.

Therapeutic
It lowers the levels of stress and anxiety by harmonizing the Pranas.

Spiritual
It induces tranquility, clarity of thought and concentration. It clears Pranic blockages and balances both nadis.

> "Calming the mind is yog.
> Not just standing on the head."
> - Swami Satchidananda

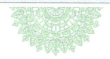

C: Suryaanuloma Viloma Pranayama

Sthiti: Vajrasana

Practice

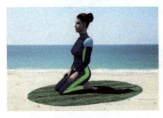
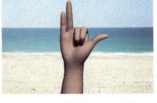
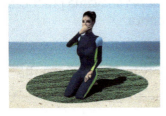

1. Adopt Nasikamudra with your right hand
2. Close the left nostril with the little and ring fingers of Nāsikāmudrā
3. Inhale and exhale slowly through the right nostril (Suryanadi) only
4. Keep the left nostril closed all the time during the practice. One cycle of inhalation and exhalation forms one round
5. Practice nine rounds

Note
1. The time taken for exhalation should be longer than for inhalation
2. To reduce fat practice this Pranayama 27 rounds before breakfast, lunch, dinner, and before sleep (4 times a day)

Limitations

For Suryanuloma-VilomaPranayama, people suffering from high blood pressure, any heart disease, and underweight problems should avoid this Practice.

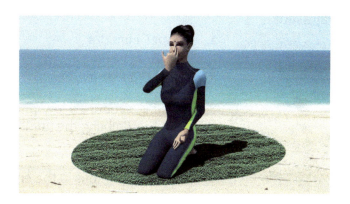

Benefits
1. This practice is useful in reducing weight
2. It increases the metabolic rate and hence burns out calories similar to physical exercise
3. This works by increasing sympathetic activation. Hence practicing this Pranayama 27 rounds 4 times a day (before breakfast, lunch, dinner and before sleep) will help you to reduce weight remarkably
4. This Pranayama is very useful as you need not find a gym or isolated place to work out to burn your calories
5. Can be done sitting anywhere, even while traveling; useful if you have pain in the legs/body which may stop you from doing your physical workouts

*"Feelings come and go like clouds in a windy sky.
Conscious breathing is my anchor."*
- Thich Nhat Hanh

D: Bhramari Pranayama

Sthiti: Vajrasana

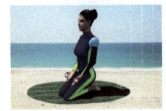

Practice

1. Adopt Cinmudrā
2. Inhale deeply
3. Exhaling, produce a low-pitched sound resembling the humming of a female bee
4. Feel the vibrations in the entire head
5. This is one round, Repeat nine rounds

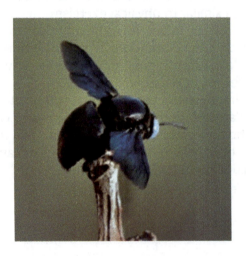

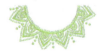

Note
1. During the Practice of Bhramari use 'N-kara' and not 'M-kara'
2. Touch the tongue to the upper (hard) palate
3. Initially, the sound vibration is felt more at the throat region only
4. With long Practices try to feel the strong vibrations in the entire head region along with its resonating effect throughout the body

Benefits

Physical
Creates a soothing effect on the nervous system. Cultures the voice and increases the melody.

Therapeutic
Relieves stress and cerebral tension. Reduces anger, anxiety, insomnia and blood pressure. Good for all psychosomatic problems as it reduces stress and tension. Eliminates throat ailments (tonsils, pains, etc.,). Speeds up the healing of tissues and so may be practiced after surgery.

Spiritual
Develop dimensional 3-D awareness. It aids in expanding the mind towards all pervasive awareness. It induces a meditative state by harmonizing the mind and directing the awareness inwards.

Limitations
Neurological and Psychiatric disorders will make patients unfit for the practice.

> *"What you think, you become."*
> - Lord Buddha

8: Dhyana

Meditation Techniques

Stress may also be responsible for increasing belly fat by triggering the adrenal glands to produce cortisol which is also known as the stress hormone. As per research, stress enhances the level of cortisol that increases the appetite which may cause belly fat. To decrease belly fat, some activities lower stress including practicing yoga meditation. Thus, if you reduce stress then it helps in lowering belly fat.

A: Nadanusardhana (A-Kāra, U- Kāra, M- Kāra, A-U-M)

A - KĀRA CHANTING

Sthiti: Vajrasana

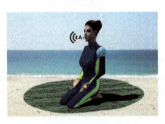

Practice

1. Sit in any meditative posture and adopt CinMudra

2. Feel completely relaxed and close your eyes

3. Inhale slowly and completely

4. While exhaling, chant 'AAA' in a low pitch

5. Feel the sound resonance in the abdomen and the lower parts of the body

6. Repeat nine times

U - KĀRA CHANTING

Sthiti: Vajrasana

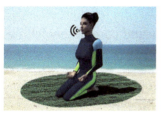

Practice

1. Sit in any meditative posture
2. Adopt CinmayaMudra
3. Feel completely relaxed and close your eyes
4. Inhale slowly and completely
5. While exhaling, chant 'UUU' in a low pitch
6. Feel the sound resonance in the chest and the middle part of the body
7. Repeat nine times

M-KĀRA CHANTING

Sthiti: Vajrasana

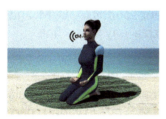

Practice

1. Sit in any meditative posture
2. Adopt AdiMudra
3. Inhale slowly and completely
4. While exhaling chant 'MMM' in a low pitch
5. Feel the sound resonance in the entire head region
6. Repeat nine times

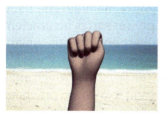

B: Om Meditation
Sthiti: Vajrasana

Practice

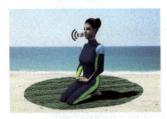

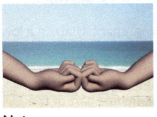

1. Sit in any meditative posture
2. Adopt Brahma Mudra
3. Inhale slowly and completely fill the lungs
4. While exhaling, chant 'A-U-M' in a low pitch
5. Feel the sound resonance through out the body
6. Repeat nine times

Note
1. Different sounds like A, U, M, and AUM are produced loudly so that they generate a fine resonance all over the body. (Resonance will occur only when the frequency of the generated sound matches the natural frequency of the body)
2. These resonant sounds act as stimulations and the post-resonance silence deepens the awareness and releases even very subtle tensions
3. Therefore, while producing different sounds (A, U, M, and AUM) try to adjust the pitch in such a way that a fine resonance is achieved

Relaxation Techniques

Relaxation keeps the whole body in proper condition. Regular practice of relaxation is useful to reduce stress & fats in various parts of our bodies. This will help to reduce weight & maintain the mind & body in proper health in the long run. As per research, insufficient sleep may also cause stress that may be responsible for weight gain. Thus, better sleep lowers depression that helps in lowering weight. Inadequate sleep also enhances the appetite which may cause an increase in weight or belly fat. So, good relaxation practices are beneficial to reduce the risk of belly fat.

9: Quick Relaxation Technique (QRT)

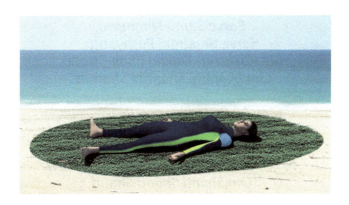

Phase I - Observing the abdominal movements
Bring your attention to the abdomen, without changing anything. Observe the movements of the abdomen.

Phase II – Associate with Breathing
Now, observe the synchronization of breathing with the movements of the abdominal wall. Now. Inhale deeply and bulge the abdomen up. While exhaling, drop down the abdomen. Practice these five rounds. While you continue the round, increase the range of movement of the abdomen. Suck the abdomen when you exhale. Enjoy the practice.

Breathing with felling
While inhaling, feel the positive energy entering the body. While exhaling, throw away all negative energy, stress, and ill- health. Maintain this feeling during the five rounds of repetition of ukara.

Phase III – Breathing with chanting
For further deep relaxation, we will chant ukara. Take a deep breath in. Feel the vibrations created by Akara in the entire abdominal cavity. Return to sitting position, Sithila dandasana Sthiti. Slowly bring the legs together. Both hands are by the side of the body. Taking support of both the elbows sit in your respective places. Both the hands are backward and the fingers facing backward. Neck relaxed. Eyes closed.

10: Closing Prayer

Om Sarve Bhavantu Sukhinah,
Sarve Santu Niramaya,
Sarve Bhadrani Pashyantu,
Ma Kashchitt Dukha Bhag Bhavet.
Om Shantihi Shantihi Shantihi.

May All Be Happy and Prosperous,
May All Be Free from Illness,
May All Life Be Auspicious,
No One Becomes a Partaker of Sorrow.
Om Shanti Shanti Shanti.

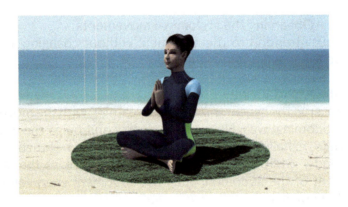

Philosophy Behind Sarve Bhavantu Sukhinah Shloka. This "Om, Sarve Bhavantu Sukhinah" means "May everyone be happy" which means that everyone, every animal, every person and every atom, energy or whatever creature should be happy and free from suffering. May all be free from diseases. May all see things auspicious. May none be subjected to misery.
Om Peace Peace Peace.

> Spiritual Growth: Pranayama practices connects the mind, body, and spirit. It encourages self-discovery and introspection, fostering a sense of purpose & inner peace.

Application of Yog Practises

KICK START

Maintain your motivation; your commitment is an investment in yourself. Establish your weight reduction goal and allocate 60 minutes each morning to kickstart your day with this yoga protocol. Follow it diligently and behold not only the changes in fat reduction but a profound transformation across all five levels of your personality.

In the present scenario, students are leading hectic lives, often stressed due to studies and competitions. Many are away from their parents, residing in hostels for higher studies. In such situations, this book serves as a boon, providing guidance for maintaining comprehensive physical, mental, emotional, and spiritual health.

Rapidly changing dietary patterns, coupled with increasingly sedentary lifestyles, expose individuals to nutrition-related non-communicable diseases, including childhood obesity.

Character and health are the cornerstones of an ideal personality. Yoga serves as a tool for the enhancement of both. Hence, prioritizing yoga is crucial, as character and health are the most vital aspects of life. By dedicating ample time to practice yoga every day and altering dietary habits, we can effectively address the growing issue of adolescent obesity.

Dear Children, this book isn't just about shedding excess fat; it's about boosting your confidence and emerging from depression. It will not only help you reduce weight, but also enhance your social interactions, making you more friendly and accomplished.

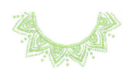

How to Achieve a Set Goal to reduce Weight?

Ready to set your weight reduction goal? Paste it somewhere visible, ensuring it stays in your focus. Transform yoga into a lifestyle.

Key elements to harness the power of visualization for weight loss:

- Sit quietly twice a day, morning and night
- Visualize your desired body shape
- Imagine people complimenting your transformation
- Visualize yourself slim – your mind shapes your reality
- Absolute focus on goals
- Time-bound efforts
- Comfort in practicing yoga
- Understanding the sequence
- A sense of self-reward, and an effortless approach
- Resolve. Decide, Determine, Discipline

As you start practicing within a month you will realize that you are feeling lighter day by day. These are key elements. Exercise is a crucial aspect of healthy living for children. Aim for a minimum of 60 minutes of yoga activity per day to prevent obesity.

Starting is simple:

- Learn techniques step by step.
- Practice the previous day's techniques before moving to new ones.
- Within fifteen days, you'll master all the techniques.
- Feel your energy levels surge.
- Track your progress:

Maintain a journal:

- Surround yourself with supportive individuals
- Seek feedback from friends, family, and well-wishers on your monthly improvements.
- Reward yourself for accomplishments.

- By tracking your progress, you may get motivated to change your eating habits
- Add online network: Try building a support network of friends and family to encourage and motivate you, or an online community where you can connect with people who have similar goals
- Post your snaps on your groups to get positive Comments which will keep motivating you to continue practises

Leverage the IAYT protocol for adolescent obesity – applicable across different stages of adolescence without hindering academic, social, or cognitive development. It cultivates a firm foundation for personality development during this critical phase. The module, encompassing various yoga paths, proves effective in addressing obesity and promoting overall adolescent development. Schools and colleges can seamlessly integrate this 60-minute routine into their timetables.

Consistent practice of IAYT can effectively manage to prevent adolescent obesity and other stress-related disorders. Yoga, as a therapeutic approach, boosts both preventive and curative effects on obesity and non-communicable diseases.

Success isn't a constant companion; setbacks are a part of the journey. Don't let challenges push you to quit midway. Stick to the protocol and incorporate the practices into your lifestyle. Over time, they'll become ingrained habits. Keep moving forward – eventually, you will cross the finishing line of your goals.

> This yog protocol is rooted in scientifically developed techniques by S-Vyasa, rigorously validated by experts, and successfully implemented in schools across Maharashtra.

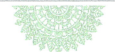

Chapter 6

Healthy and Balanced Eating Habits

What we eat plays a significant role in our mental and emotional wellbeing. By making mindful choices about our diet and incorporating healthy, nourishing foods, we can improve our mood, energy levels, and overall outlook on life.

Sadguru, an Indian spiritual leader, has emphasized the importance of mindful eating and its impact on our overall well-being. He states, "When you eat, you are not just consuming food - you are taking in the energy of the food and the environment around you. Your body is like a temple, and the food you consume should be treated with respect."

As Sadguru states, "When you eat well, you think well."

The next part of the book focuses on how to set good eating habits and have a balanced diet that can help the child develop improved health, better academic performance, a strong work ethic, and improved social skills and increased self-confidence.

> *Empower children to love their bodies, not with excess weight, but by developing eating habits for strength*

Out of Sight, Out of Mind

In a world bustling with distractions and temptations, the age-old adage "out of sight, out of mind" holds a significant place. This simple yet profound phrase encapsulates a psychological principle that influences our behaviors, decisions, and habits more than we often realize. Whether we're discussing decluttering our physical space, managing our digital lives, or even fostering healthier eating habits, the concept of "out of sight, out of mind" can guide us toward making better choices and leading more intentional lives.

At its core, "out of sight, out of mind" speaks to the human tendency to prioritize what's immediately visible or accessible. When something is no longer within our visual or mental reach, it tends to fade from our thoughts and considerations. This phenomenon is deeply rooted in the way our brains process information and allocate cognitive resources. In essence, if we can't see or easily recall something, it becomes less likely to occupy our mental space

One domain where this principle shines is in the realm of eating habits, particularly the battle against mindless snacking on unhealthy foods. The allure of junk food can be overwhelming, especially when it's prominently displayed or stored within arm's reach. But here's where the power of "out of sight, out of mind" comes into play.

James Clear, renowned author and expert on habit formation, delves into this phenomenon in his best-selling book "Atomic Habits." Clear suggests that rather than solely relying on willpower to resist temptations, we can engineer our environment to align with our desired behaviors. He advocates for shaping our surroundings in ways that encourage positive actions and discourage detrimental ones. The idea is not to test the limits of our self-control but to strategically set up our environment to make healthy choices the path of least resistance.

The implications of "out of sight, out of mind" extend beyond personal habits and into the realm of parenting and child development. Parents play a pivotal role in shaping their children's behaviors and attitudes, especially when it comes to food choices. Children are highly impressionable and often mimic the behaviors they observe in their caregivers.

Imagine you have a weakness for ice cream and chocolates, and you find it hard to resist these treats when they are readily available in your kitchen. Every time you open your freezer or pantry, you see these sugary indulgences, and you're often tempted to consume them, even when you're not genuinely hungry. To improve your eating habits and make it easier to choose healthier options, you decide not to keep ice cream and chocolates at home. Instead, you stock your kitchen with a variety of fresh fruits, vegetables, and other nutritious snacks. With this change, you've made it "out of sight" when it comes to ice cream and chocolates. When cravings strike, you'd have to make a conscious effort to go out and buy these treats. This extra step introduces a barrier to access, which can deter impulsive consumption.

Over time, you'll notice a significant difference in your eating habits. You are more likely to opt for the available healthier snacks because they are "in sight." When you want a snack, you'll grab an apple or some carrot sticks instead of reaching for the ice cream that's no longer within easy reach. By making these changes and keeping unhealthy options "out of sight" at home, you're creating an environment that promotes better eating habits and makes it easier to choose nutritious foods. This simple adjustment can help you align your home environment with your health and wellness goals.

What You as a Parent Eat is What Your Child Would Want to Eat

Parents play a critical role in shaping the behavior, habits, and attitudes of their children. This is especially true when it comes to food and nutrition. As a parent, the food choices you make and the daily food you have has a profound impact on your child's eating habits and preferences. Children are more likely to try new foods and develop healthy eating habits if they see their parents doing the same. If you want your child to eat a healthy and balanced diet, it is important to lead by example. As a parent, you should make an effort to eat a variety of fruits, vegetables, whole grains, and lean proteins and limit processed and high-fat foods intake.

If parents consistently indulge in junk food and unhealthy snacks in front of their children, it sends a conflicting message. While verbal instructions might emphasize the importance of nutritious eating, actions speak louder than words. By adopting the principle of "out of sight, out of mind," parents can create an environment that fosters healthy eating habits. This involves not only keeping junk food hidden but also actively promoting and enjoying nutritious options. When children are surrounded by wholesome foods and witness their parents making mindful choices, these behaviors become ingrained and serve as a foundation for a lifetime of wellness.

If the parents want to cultivate a positive attitude towards food in the children, the children need to see their parents enjoying their meals and taking the time to savor and appreciate the flavors and textures of different foods. By modeling healthy eating habits, parents can help their children develop a healthy relationship with food and avoid the pitfalls of fad diets, disordered eating, and obesity. Parents can not just model healthy eating habits, they can also involve their children in meal planning and preparation. This can help children develop a sense of ownership and pride in the food choices they make and it will encourage them to try new foods and flavors.

I have consciously made an effort to have a simple diet, keeping in mind that I can share whatever is on my plate with my child and it has been an amazing journey so far. I encourage parents to make conscious choices about their own diet and to eat in a way that is healthy and balanced. This will not only benefit the parents' own health, but will also set a positive example for their children to follow and as a family it will develop lifelong habits of healthy eating and nutrition.

The phrase "out of sight, out of mind" highlights the idea that when something is not visible or easily accessible, it becomes less likely to be thought about or indulged in.

As parents, it is crucial to create an environment that promotes healthy eating habits for children. If a parent regularly indulges in junk food, the child may want to eat the same by imitating them. By keeping junk food out of sight, parents help create a nutrition rich environment in their homes for their children and help them develop good habits for life.

> *Your child's life is your responsibility*

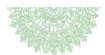

Create an Environment to Create Good Habits

Yes, creating good eating habits, such as eating on time and in a specific place, can have many benefits for children's development and well-being. Consistently eating meals at the same time and in a designated area can help establish a routine and promote a sense of structure in a child's life.

Additionally, eating in a specific place can help minimize distractions and encourage mindfulness while eating. This can promote better digestion and absorption of nutrients, as well as help children develop healthy eating habits that can benefit them throughout their lives.

I was recently at a friend's house for dinner. We were all sitting around talking, reminiscing about the good old days. My friend's wife interrupted our conversation with a "dinner call." We all stood up and went to our seats at the dinner table. We all started eating, but I noticed that my friend's child was not interested in dinner at all. After a few minutes, his mother got up, led him to the living room, turned on the TV, and began watching his favorite cartoon show before he began eating. When the child was very young, he was fed in front of the television! When he was old enough to eat on his own and cartoons entered his life, Pokemon and Doraemon were his constant dinner companions. What began as yet another thing, had now become a habit. To keep up with his dinner, he needed cartoons or anything on TV!

But here's an interesting question: if the kid's parents can have a proper dinner place away from digital distractions, why can't he? And the answer is Habit!!

A small set of a behavior that, if unnoticed, becomes a pattern. When we realize it has become a habit, it is perhaps a little late.

We as parents frequently fail to recognize that whatever habits our children ingrain, good or bad, we are responsible for it. Take, for example, my friend and his wife, who initially believed that having dinner is more important than where you have it and now facing a mammoth task of reducing the screen time during the dinner for their kid.. All of these small situations eventually add up to form a pattern. But how do we, as parents and relatives, deal with this issue?

First and foremost, we must recognize that our smallest actions are leading to the formation of patterns. We must be disciplined while dealing with our children. And by discipline, I mean having a designated area where you can all eat together, putting only the foods on your plate that you want your child to eat, and most importantly, having a routine so that you can eat meals on time. All of these small things add up to form a large thing known as a habit!

Habit, - which, if not addressed in the early stages, can cause problems. Habits - which now make my friend's child's behavior appear bizarre? When we let them enjoy their meals in front of the TV or while watching something over the internet it imprints on their mind that it is good behavior.

Furthermore, establishing healthy habits around food and mealtime can also have a positive impact on other areas of a child's life, such as their sleep schedule and overall mood. It can also help them understand the importance of discipline and consistency in achieving goals and maintaining a healthy lifestyle.

James Clear, the author of "Atomic Habits", emphasizes the importance of creating an environment that supports healthy habits. He believes that our habits are largely a product of our environment, and that we can make it easier to build good habits and break bad ones by making small changes to our surroundings. In his book, he writes:

"You do not rise to the level of your goals. You fall to the level of your systems. What you do every day matters more than what you do once in a while. If you want to build better habits, you need to change your environment."

Clear suggests that we can make small changes to our environment that will make it easier to stick to healthy habits. For example, if you want to eat more fruits and vegetables, you could make sure that you always have them on hand by keeping a bowl of fresh fruit on your kitchen counter. If you want to drink more water, you could keep a water bottle on your desk or carry one with you wherever you go.

Clear also emphasizes the importance of starting small when creating new habits. He suggests focusing on making small, incremental changes to your behavior rather than trying to make drastic changes all at once. Over time, these small changes will add up and lead to significant improvements in your health and overall well-being.

I can provide examples of how habit creation helped individuals become successful in their fields.

One example is Magnus Carlsen, a Norwegian chess grandmaster who became the world chess champion in 2013 at the age of 22. Carlsen's father introduced him to chess when he was just five years old, and he quickly became obsessed with the game. From a young age, Carlsen developed a daily habit of playing and studying chess for several hours a day. He also played against other chess players, including his older sister, and participated in local chess tournaments.

Carlsen's daily habit of playing and studying chess helped him develop his skills and become one of the best chess players in the world. He continued to refine his approach to chess throughout his career, using technology to study his opponents and analyze his own games. By making chess a daily habit, Carlsen was able to achieve his goal of becoming a world champion.

To summarize, I'd like to quote James Clear,

"Habits are like the atoms of our lives, each one is a fundamental unit that contributes to your overall improvement."

The onus is on us to ensure that we want our children to grow up well.

Eat Mindfully: It Can Help You in Day-to-Day Life

Overall, good eating habits can help children develop a strong foundation for a successful and fulfilling future.

We often hear about the importance of eating a healthy diet for our future health, but what about the benefits of eating mindfully for our present well-being? Mindful eating is a practice that involves paying attention to the experience of eating, without judgment or distraction. By focusing on the sensory experience of eating, we can enhance our enjoyment of food, improve our digestion, and reduce stress and anxiety.

One of the biggest benefits of mindful eating is that it helps us develop a more positive relationship with food. Many of us have a complicated relationship with food, where we may feel guilty or ashamed after eating certain foods, or feel like we have to restrict ourselves in order to maintain a certain body shape. Mindful eating encourages us to let go of these negative associations with food, and instead approach eating with a sense of curiosity and openness.

Eating mindfully can also improve our digestion. When we eat in a rush or while distracted, we may not chew our food properly, which can lead to digestive issues like bloating and discomfort. By taking the time to savor each bite and chew our food thoroughly, we can help our bodies digest our food more efficiently.

Finally, mindful eating can help reduce stress and anxiety. When we eat while distracted or rushed, our bodies can go into a stress response, which can interfere with digestion and overall well-being. By taking the time to slow down and focus on our food, we can activate our parasympathetic nervous system, which helps our bodies rest and digest.

Sadhguru, an Indian yogi, mystic, and author, emphasizes the importance of living in the present moment and being fully present for each breath. In his book, "Inner Engineering: A Yogi's Guide to Joy," he writes, "One breath in and one breath out is one unit of your life. If you learn to live this one breath fully, you will know the fullness of life."

A healthy and balanced diet is crucial for the development of a child, especially during the age of 0 to 5, which is a critical period for growth and development. During this time, the body is rapidly developing, and the brain is also developing at a remarkable pace, which makes proper nutrition essential.

Research suggests that a balanced diet consisting of a variety of nutrients such as proteins, carbohydrates, healthy fats, vitamins, and minerals is important for the development of the brain, bones, muscles, and overall growth of a child. A diet that lacks essential nutrients can lead to stunted growth, weak bones, cognitive deficits, and other health problems.

Moreover, a balanced diet is not only important for physical growth but also for cognitive and emotional development. A well-nourished child is more likely to have better cognitive abilities, perform better academically, and have a lower risk of developing behavioral and emotional problems.

Additionally, unhealthy diets during early childhood can have long-term consequences on a child's health. Children who are exposed to unhealthy diets during their early years are more likely to develop chronic diseases such as obesity, diabetes, and heart diseases later in life.

Therefore, parents and caregivers must provide children with a healthy and balanced diet from an early age to ensure their optimal growth and development. It is essential to offer a variety of foods to children and to limit their intake of processed and sugary foods. By doing so, we can lay the foundation for a healthy and happy life for our children.

Your Food is a Need and Not a Want

Eating simple food that our body can easily digest can have numerous benefits for our overall health and well-being. When we consume food that takes a lot of time to digest, it can lead to a lack of focus and energy, which can have a negative impact on our productivity, studies, and hobbies.

The first step towards achieving maximum results with minimum efforts is to avoid all artificial sugar, refined flour, processed and packaged food. These types of food are often high in calories, unhealthy fats, and sugars, and lack essential nutrients that our body needs to function properly. Consuming such foods can lead to a slowing down of our body and add lethargy, making us feel tired and sluggish.

When we consume simple, whole foods that are easy to digest, such as fruits, vegetables, whole grains, lean proteins, and healthy fats, our body can quickly absorb the nutrients, providing us with a steady source of energy throughout the day. These foods are rich in essential vitamins, minerals, and fiber, which are vital for maintaining good health and preventing diseases.

Furthermore, eating simple food can help us develop a healthy relationship with food. Food is not a luxury but a source of energy that our body needs to function correctly. By treating food as a basic need rather than a want, we can make healthier choices and avoid overindulging in unhealthy foods that can have adverse effects on our health. In Ayurveda, an ancient system of medicine from India, foods are categorized into three types: Sattvic, Rajasic, and Tamasic, based on their effect on the mind and body.

Sattvic foods are considered pure, clean, and wholesome, and are believed to promote mental clarity, tranquility, and spiritual growth. Examples of Sattvic foods include fresh fruits and vegetables, nuts, seeds, whole grains, and dairy products.

Rajasic foods are believed to be stimulating and energizing, but also agitating and distracting. Examples of Rajasic foods include spicy or pungent foods, caffeine, and processed foods.

Tamasic foods are considered heavy, dull, and inert, and are believed to promote lethargy, inertia, and negativity. Examples of Tamasic foods include meat, alcohol, processed or stale foods, and artificially flavored foods.

In general, Sadhguru recommends avoiding Tamasic foods as they are believed to have a negative impact on both physical and mental health. He advises eating a Sattvic diet, which is believed to be the most conducive for spiritual growth and overall well-being.

Sadhguru once said, "The food you eat can either be the safest and most powerful form of medicine or the slowest form of poison." This quote emphasizes the importance of paying attention to what we eat and how it affects our health. By instilling healthy eating habits in children, we can help them cultivate a positive relationship with food and set them up for a healthy and fulfilling future.

To Conclude, Good eating habits play a crucial role in shaping a future. While it's important to live in the present and enjoy every moment, having good eating habits and being mindful of what we eat is not contrary to that philosophy. In fact, it can enhance our ability to fully enjoy and make the most of each moment. Here's how it aligns with the idea of living in the present:

1. **Immediate Benefits:** Good eating habits can provide immediate benefits such as increased energy, better focus, and improved mood. When you're feeling physically and mentally well, you're more likely to be present in the moment and fully engage with your activities and experiences.

2. **Long-Term Well-Being:** While the present moment is important, we also have a responsibility to care for our future selves. By maintaining good eating habits, we invest in our long-term health and quality of life, ensuring that we can continue to enjoy life to the fullest as we age.

3. **Preventing Health Issues:** Good eating habits can help prevent chronic health issues that could otherwise detract from the quality of your life in the future. This means fewer doctor's visits, medications, and potential health-related stress.

4. **Balanced Approach:** Good eating habits don't necessarily mean restrictive or joyless eating. It's about balance. You can savor delicious, nutritious foods and enjoy occasional treats without guilt. This balanced approach allows you to appreciate the present while caring for your long-term well-being.

5. **Enhanced Physical and Mental Resilience:** Proper nutrition can help your body and mind better cope with stress and challenges in the present, allowing you to navigate life's ups and downs more effectively.

6. **Building Healthy Rituals:** Developing good eating habits can be a form of self-care and mindfulness. Preparing and enjoying nutritious meals can become a ritual that helps you appreciate the process and the flavors in the present.

In essence, good eating habits support a holistic approach to well-being, which includes both the enjoyment of the present and the cultivation of a healthy future. It's about finding a balance that allows you to fully embrace each moment while taking steps to ensure you can continue doing so in the future.

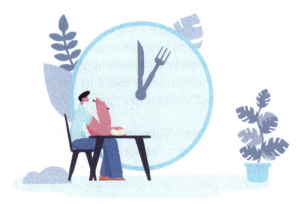

Vital Tips on What to Eat and Not to Eat

As a professional in the creative field, I understand the importance of nurturing both body and mind. Just as creativity knows no bounds, our well-being too shouldn't be confined. It's not just about what we create with our hands, but also what we fuel our bodies and souls with.

In the symphony of creation, a healthy lifestyle becomes the melody that resonates most harmoniously. Remember, in the realm of creativity, a healthy body and a nourished soul are the greatest assets, shaping not just our work but our entire journey. So, let's paint our lives with the vibrant hues of health and wellness, crafting masterpieces both inside and out.

Understanding what to eat and what to avoid is crucial for maintaining a balanced diet. As the saying goes, "Let food be thy medicine, and medicine be thy food" – a wisdom imparted by Hippocrates, emphasizing the profound impact of nutrition on our overall well-being. It's essential to acknowledge that individual dietary requirements differ, and seeking guidance from a licensed healthcare professional or registered dietitian is vital for personalized nutrition advice. Just as one size doesn't fit all in clothing, comprehending your body's needs is vital to creating a tailored diet plan.

Below, I've shared my personal diet, which has significantly contributed to my overall development. Please understand that this is not a prescription but merely provided for your information. It's important to customize your diet based on your unique body and health needs. Remember, your body is a temple; nourish it with the right foods and watch it flourish.

Always Stay Hydrated

Drinking a glass of water every hour can have several benefits for the body, including:

1. **Staying hydrated:** Drinking water throughout the day helps to maintain the body's hydration levels, which is important for overall health.

2. **Improving digestion:** Water helps to flush out toxins and waste products from the body, which can improve digestion and prevent constipation.

3. **Boosting energy levels:** Dehydration can cause fatigue and sluggishness, so drinking water regularly can help to keep energy levels up.

4. **Supporting kidney function:** Drinking enough water can help to keep the kidneys functioning properly, which is important for removing waste products from the body.

5. **Maintaining healthy skin:** Drinking water can help to keep the skin hydrated and prevent dryness, which can improve its appearance.

However, it's important to note that everyone's water needs may vary depending on factors such as age, activity level, and climate. It's recommended to drink enough water to keep your urine a pale yellow color throughout the day, and to consult with a healthcare professional if you have any concerns about your water intake.

> Hereditary tendencies & family influences on eating habits play a vital role.

Importance of Sleep

The importance of sleep and the benefits it can bring to our physical, mental, and spiritual well-being. Some of the benefits of sleeping according to Sadhguru are:

1. **Rejuvenation of the Body:** Sleep allows our body to recover and repair itself from the wear and tear of daily life. It is during sleep that our cells regenerate and our immune system strengthens, helping us fight off illnesses and diseases.

2. **Improved Brain Function:** Sleep is crucial for brain function and cognitive processes. It helps consolidate memories, enhances learning, and improves overall mental alertness.

3. **Better Emotional Balance:** Lack of sleep can lead to emotional instability and mood swings. Adequate sleep, on the other hand, promotes emotional balance, reducing the risk of anxiety and depression.

4. **Increased Energy and Vitality:** Quality sleep is essential for energy restoration and vitality. It helps us feel refreshed and recharged, ready to face the challenges of the day ahead.

5. **Spiritual Well-being:** According to Sadhguru, sleep is not just a physical necessity but also a spiritual practice. It can help us connect with our inner self, access deeper levels of consciousness and enhance our spiritual growth.

> *Man gets the energy directly when he feeds on vegetables & fruits as they are the primary producers.*

Consuming Ghee Before a Meal

Sadhguru, a spiritual leader and yoga guru, has spoken about the benefits of consuming ghee before a meal. According to him, there are some advantages to eating ghee before a meal. Promotes digestion: Ghee stimulates the secretion of digestive juices in the stomach, which can aid in digestion. It also helps in the absorption of fat-soluble vitamins and minerals.

1. **Boosts metabolism:** Ghee is rich in butyric acid, which helps improve metabolism and digestion. This can lead to better energy levels and improved overall health.

2. **Supports healthy weight management:** Contrary to popular belief, ghee can actually aid in weight loss. It helps the body burn fat more efficiently, leading to a healthier weight.

3. **Supports a healthy immune system:** Ghee is rich in antioxidants and vitamins A, D, E, and K, which are essential for maintaining a healthy immune system.

4. **Promotes mental clarity:** Ghee contains omega-3 and omega-9 fatty acids, which are essential for brain function. Consuming ghee before a meal can help improve mental clarity and focus.

It's worth noting that while ghee can have some health benefits, it is also high in calories and should be consumed in moderation. Additionally, those with dairy allergies or lactose intolerance should avoid consuming ghee.

> *By eating many fruits and vegetables in place of fast food and junk food, people could avoid obesity.*

Protein

Protein is an essential macronutrient that is necessary for the growth & repair of tissues in the body. It is made up of amino acids, which are the building blocks of protein. Some benefits of consuming protein include:

1. **Muscle growth and repair:** Protein is essential for building and repairing muscle tissue.

2. **Improved satiety:** Protein helps you feel full and satisfied, which can lead to a reduction in overall calorie intake.

3. **Increased metabolism:** Protein has a higher thermic effect than carbohydrates or fat, which means that your body burns more calories carbohydrates or fat, which means that your body burns more calories digesting protein than it does digesting other macronutrients.

4. **Improved immune function:** Protein is necessary for the production of antibodies & other immune system components.

5. **Better bone health:** Adequate protein intake can help prevent bone loss and reduce the risk of osteoporosis.

However, Sadhguru also stresses the importance of consuming protein from natural sources, such as whole grains, nuts, seeds, and legumes, rather than from processed or animal-based sources. He has advocated for a plant-based diet that is rich in protein, as well as other essential nutrients. According to Sadhguru's hack on protein from soaked groundnuts and bananas, he suggests soaking groundnuts for a few hours and then blending them with bananas to make a protein-rich shake. While this may provide some protein, it is important to note that groundnuts & bananas are not complete sources of protein and may not provide all the essential amino acids needed for optimal health.

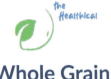

Whole Grains

Choose whole grains such as brown rice, quinoa, and oats instead of refined grains. Whole grains are a good source of fiber and help regulate blood sugar levels. Whole grains are an important part of a healthy diet and are rich in nutrients such as fiber, vitamins, and minerals. Here are some of the benefits of incorporating whole grains into your diet:

1. **Improved digestive health:** Whole grains are an excellent source of fiber, which can help regulate bowel movements and prevent constipation.

2. **Reduced risk of chronic diseases:** Studies have shown that consuming whole grains can reduce the risk of developing chronic diseases such as heart disease, stroke, and type 2 diabetes.

3. **Better weight management:** Whole grains can help you feel full for longer periods of time, which can help you manage your weight.

4. **Lower cholesterol levels:** Eating whole grains may help lower levels of LDL or "bad" cholesterol, which can reduce your risk of heart disease.

5. **Improved brain function:** Whole grains contain vitamins and minerals that are important for brain function, such as B vitamins and iron.

> *Elevate your child's health with whole grains - nature's gift for a strong, smart, and happy future. Feed their bodies, nourish their minds, and watch them thrive!*

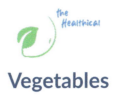

Vegetables

Eat a variety of vegetables, including leafy greens, cruciferous vegetables, and colorful vegetables. Vegetables are rich in vitamins, minerals, and antioxidants that support overall health. Here are some of the main benefits:

1. **Nutrient density:** Vegetables are packed with essential vitamins, minerals, and nutrients that our bodies need to function properly. Eating a variety of fresh vegetables ensures that you get a diverse array of nutrients that support overall health and wellness.

2. **Fiber:** Vegetables are a rich source of fiber, which helps promote healthy digestion and prevents constipation. Fiber also helps regulate blood sugar levels and can reduce the risk of developing certain chronic diseases such as heart disease, diabetes, and cancer.

3. **Hydration:** Many vegetables have a high water content, which can help keep the body hydrated and support healthy skin and hair.

4. **Antioxidants:** Fresh vegetables are rich in antioxidants, which are compounds that help protect the body against damage from free radicals. Free radicals can contribute to chronic inflammation and disease, so getting a variety of antioxidants from fresh vegetables can help protect against these harmful effects.

5. **Weight management:** Eating fresh vegetables can help support weight management by providing low-calorie, nutrient dense options that keep you feeling full and satisfied. This can help prevent overeating and reduce the risk of obesity.

Overall, eating fresh vegetables is an essential part of a healthy diet and can provide a wide range of health benefits for the body.

Fruits

Eat a variety of fruits, including seasonal fruits. Fruits are a good source of fiber, vitamins, and minerals. Eating fruits is beneficial for our overall health and well-being. Here are some of the benefits of eating fruits:

1. **Rich in nutrients:** Fruits are rich in vitamins, minerals, fiber, and antioxidants. These nutrients are essential for our body to function properly and to prevent various diseases.

2. **Helps in digestion:** Fruits contain natural enzymes that aid in digestion and improve bowel movement. Eating fruits on an empty stomach can help cleanse the digestive tract and promote better digestion.

3. **Boosts immunity:** Fruits contain a variety of vitamins and antioxidants that can help boost our immune system and protect us from infections and diseases.

4. **Good for skin and hair:** Fruits contain essential vitamins and minerals that promote healthy skin and hair. Eating fruits regularly can help reduce wrinkles, prevent acne, and promote hair growth.

When to eat fruits:
According to Sadhguru, the best time to eat fruits is on an empty stomach, preferably in the morning. This is because the natural sugars in fruits are easily absorbed by the body and provide an instant energy boost. Eating fruits on an empty stomach can also help cleanse the digestive tract and promote better digestion. It is important to eat fruits in moderation and to choose a variety of fruits to get a wide range of nutrients.

Nuts and Seeds

Nuts and seeds are nutrient-dense foods that can provide many health benefits when consumed as part of a healthy diet. Include nuts and seeds in your diet for healthy fats and protein. They are also a good source of vitamins and minerals. Here are some of the benefits of eating nuts and seeds:

1. **Rich in healthy fats:** Nuts and seeds are rich in mono - unsaturated and polyunsaturated fats, which are healthy fats that can help lower cholesterol levels and reduce the risk of heart disease.

2. **High in protein:** Nuts and seeds are also high in protein, which is essential for building and repairing tissues in the body.

3. **Good source of fiber:** Nuts and seeds are a good source of dietary fiber, which can help improve digestion, regulate blood sugar levels, and promote feelings of fullness.

4. **Rich in vitamins and minerals:** Nuts and seeds are also rich in vitamins and minerals, such as vitamin E, magnesium, and zinc, which are important for overall health and well-being.

5. **May reduce the risk of chronic diseases:** Studies have shown that eating nuts and seeds regularly may help reduce the risk of chronic diseases, such as heart disease, diabetes, and certain types of cancer.

6. **Versatile and easy to incorporate into your diet:** Nuts and seeds are easy to add to your diet as a snack, ingredient in meals or topping on dishes.

Overall, including a variety of nuts and seeds in your diet can provide many health benefits and may help improve your overall well-being.

Legumes

Include legumes such as lentils, chickpeas, and beans in your diet for protein, fiber, and micronutrients. Legumes, such as lentils, beans, chickpeas, and peas, are an excellent source of plant-based protein, fiber, vitamins, and minerals. Here are some benefits of including legumes in your diet:

1. **High in protein:** Legumes are an excellent source of plant-based protein. They provide a complete source of protein when combined with grains like rice or wheat.

2. **Rich in fiber:** Legumes are high in dietary fiber, which promotes healthy digestion, lowers cholesterol levels, and reduces the risk of heart disease.

3. **Low glycemic index:** Legumes have a low glycemic index, which means they cause a gradual increase in blood sugar levels, preventing sudden spikes and crashes.

4. **Source of vitamins and minerals:** Legumes are a good source of vitamins and minerals, including folate, iron, potassium, and magnesium.

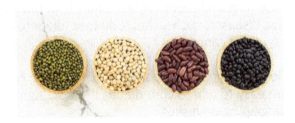

Spices

Use spices such as turmeric, cumin, & ginger to add flavor & health benefits to your meals. Spices have anti-inflammatory & antioxidant properties. They are not only used to add flavor & aroma to dishes, but also have a number of health benefits. Here are some of the benefits of spices:

1. **Antioxidant properties:** Many spices such as turmeric, cinnamon, & cloves contain high levels of antioxidants which help protect against cellular damage caused by free radicals.

2. **Anti-inflammatory properties:** Spices like ginger, garlic, & cumin are known for their anti-inflammatory properties which can help reduce inflammation in the body & improve health.

3. **Improved digestion:** Spices like black pepper, cumin, & fennel help improve digestion by stimulating the production of digestive enzymes, reducing inflammation in the gut, & promoting the growth of beneficial gut bacteria.

4. **Boost immunity:** Many spices such as turmeric, ginger, & cinnamon contain compounds that can help boost the immune system, protecting the body against infections & diseases.

5. **Weight loss:** Spices like cayenne pepper, ginger, & cinnamon can help boost metabolism, reduce appetite, & promote fat burning, which can aid in weight loss.

6. **Lower blood sugar levels:** Certain spices like cinnamon, turmeric, & fenugreek have been found to help regulate blood sugar levels in people with diabetes.

Overall, incorporating a variety of spices into your diet can provide numerous health benefits & add flavor & interest to your meals

Eating Breakfast

Eating a healthy breakfast provides a number of benefits for our bodies and minds. Here are some of the main benefits:

1. **Boosts metabolism:** Breakfast helps to kick-start your metabolism, which is important for burning calories throughout the day.

2. **Provides energy:** A healthy breakfast can provide us with the energy we need to start the day off on the right foot, and keep us energized until our next meal.

3. **Helps with weight management:** People who eat a healthy breakfast tend to consume fewer calories throughout the day, which can help with weight management.

4. **Improves cognitive function:** Breakfast provides the brain with the nutrients it needs to function at its best, which can improve memory, concentration, and overall cognitive performance.

5. **Reduces the risk of chronic diseases:** Eating a healthy breakfast can help reduce the risk of chronic diseases such as heart disease, diabetes, and obesity.

6. **Improves mood:** Starting the day off with a healthy breakfast can help improve our mood and reduce feelings of stress and anxiety.

Overall, eating a healthy breakfast is an important part of maintaining a healthy lifestyle and can provide numerous benefits for our bodies and minds.

Please Note: I suggest avoiding following foods & habits that I believe are harmful to the body and mind.

Processed and Packaged Foods

Children should avoid processed foods because their bodies and brains are still developing, and need a healthy, balanced diet to support their growth and development.

Here are some of the reasons for avoiding processed foods for children:

1. **Lack of nutrients:** Processed foods are often low in essential nutrients, such as vitamins, minerals, and fiber, that growing children need for optimal health and development.

2. **High in sugar and unhealthy fats:** Many processed foods are high in added sugars and unhealthy fats, which can contribute to obesity, diabetes, and other health problems in children.

3. **Negative impact on cognitive development:** A diet that is high in processed foods can have a negative impact on cognitive development in children, leading to poor academic performance and behavioral problems.

4. **Addictive properties:** Processed foods often contain addictive substances such as sugar, salt, and artificial flavorings, which can make it difficult for children to develop healthy eating habits.

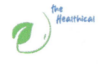

Artificial Sugar

Artificial sweeteners are synthetic sugar substitutes that are often used in place of sugar to reduce calorie intake or to provide sweetness without raising blood sugar levels. While they are generally considered safe for consumption in moderate amounts, some studies have raised concerns about their potential health effects.

Here are some potential benefits of avoiding artificial sugar:

1. **Improved blood sugar control:** Artificial sweeteners are often used by people with diabetes as a sugar substitute. However, some studies suggest that consuming artificial sweeteners may still have an impact on blood sugar levels and insulin response. Avoiding artificial sugar altogether may help to better regulate blood sugar levels.

2. **Reduced risk of weight gain and obesity:** Some studies have suggested that consuming artificial sweeteners may be associated with weight gain and obesity. By avoiding artificial sugar and choosing natural, whole foods instead, individuals may be able to better manage their weight and reduce their risk of obesity.

3. **Improved gut health:** Some research has suggested that artificial sweeteners may disrupt the balance of bacteria in the gut, which could have negative impacts on digestive health. By avoiding artificial sugar, individuals may be able to support a healthier gut microbiome.

It is important to note that natural sugars found in fruits, vegetables, and whole foods are still an important part of a balanced diet and should not be eliminated entirely.

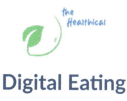

Digital Eating

Eating while watching TV or using a phone or other digital device is often referred to as "distracted eating" or "digital eating."

Here are some potential benefits of avoiding this behavior:

1. **Better digestion:** When we are distracted while eating, we eat faster and may not chew our food as thoroughly. This can make it more difficult for our digestive system to break down the food properly, which can lead to digestive discomfort such as bloating and indigestion. By avoiding distracted eating, we can improve our digestion and reduce these symptoms.

2. **Improved mindfulness:** Mindful eating involves paying attention to the experience of eating, including the taste, texture, and smell of the food, as well as our hunger and fullness cues. When we eat while distracted, we may not be fully aware of these sensations, which can lead to overeating and poor food choices. By avoiding distracted eating, we can improve our mindfulness around food and make healthier choices.

3. **Reduced risk of weight gain:** Studies have shown that people who eat while watching TV or using a phone or other digital device tend to consume more calories and are more likely to be overweight or obese. By avoiding distracted eating, we can reduce our calorie intake and reduce our risk of weight gain.

4. **Improved enjoyment of food:** When we are fully present and mindful while eating, we can more fully enjoy the experience of eating and appreciate the flavors and textures of the food. By avoiding distracted eating, we can improve our relationship with food and develop a greater appreciation for the nourishment it provides.

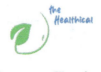

Stress Eating

Stress eating, also known as emotional eating, is a common behavior where people turn to food as a way to cope with stress, anxiety, or other negative emotions.

Here are some potential benefits of avoiding stress eating:

1. **Improved mental health:** While stress eating may provide temporary relief from negative emotions, it can also contribute to feelings of guilt, shame, and self-judgment. By avoiding stress eating, individuals can develop healthier coping mechanisms for managing stress and improve their overall mental health.

2. **Better weight management:** Stress eating often involves consuming high-calorie, high-fat, or sugary foods, which can lead to weight gain and obesity. By avoiding stress eating, individuals can better manage their calorie intake and maintain a healthy weight.

3. **Improved physical health:** Consuming unhealthy foods as a way to cope with stress can contribute to a range of health problems, including heart disease, high blood pressure, and diabetes. By avoiding stress eating and choosing healthier foods, individuals can improve their overall physical health.

4. **Increased self-awareness:** Avoiding stress eating requires individuals to become more self-aware of their emotional state and learn healthier coping mechanisms. By developing this self-awareness, individuals can improve their overall emotional intelligence and become better equipped to manage stress in a healthy way.

Alcohol

Alcohol consumption can have a negative impact on our physical and mental health, as well as our spiritual growth.

Here are some of the reasons for avoiding alcohol:

1. **Harmful to the body:** Alcohol is a toxic substance that can damage our internal organs, including the liver and brain. It can also weaken the immune system and make us more susceptible to diseases.

2. **Impacts our mental state:** Alcohol can impair our judgment, memory, and decision-making abilities. It can also lead to mood swings and depression.

3. **Hinders spiritual growth:** According to Sadhguru, alcohol consumption can block our spiritual growth by clouding our awareness and inhibiting our ability to experience higher levels of consciousness.

4. **Addiction:** Alcohol has addictive properties, and regular consumption can lead to dependence and withdrawal symptoms.

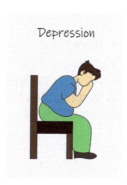

Non-Vegetarian Food

Non-vegetarian food can have a negative impact on human development, both physically and spiritually. Sadhguru, gives reasons to avoid non-vegetarian food in his book "Inner Engineering: A Yogi's Guide to Joy".

Here are a few reasons he gives for avoiding non-vegetarian food:

1. **Energy levels:** Non-vegetarian food is "heavy" and takes a lot of energy to digest. This can leave individuals feeling tired and lethargic, and can negatively impact their overall energy levels.

2. **Mind and emotions:** Non-vegetarian food can create an imbalance in the mind and emotions, leading to negative thought patterns and behaviors. He argues that a plant-based diet can promote greater mental clarity and emotional stability.

3. **Karma:** Non-vegetarian food involves taking on the karma of the animal that was killed. This can create negative karmic consequences and block spiritual growth.

4. **Health:** Some individuals may need to consume non-vegetaran food for specific health reasons, he suggests that a plant-based diet can be just as nutritious and offer a range of health benefits.

Overall, I encourage individuals to avoid non-vegetarian food in order to promote physical health, mental clarity, emotional stability, and spiritual growth. I suggest that a plant-based diet can be a more holistic and sustainable choice for individuals looking to live a healthier and more fulfilling life.

Gluten

Gluten is a protein found in wheat, barley, and rye. Some people are unable to tolerate gluten due to a medical condition called celiac disease, which is an autoimmune disorder that causes the body to react to gluten and damage the small intestine. Other people may have a sensitivity or intolerance to gluten, which can cause symptoms such as bloating, abdominal pain, and diarrhea.

Here are some potential benefits that have been associated with a gluten-free diet:

1. **Improved digestive symptoms:** Some people may experience improved digestive symptoms, such as bloating, gas, and diarrhea, when they eliminate gluten from their diet. This may be due to the fact that gluten can be difficult to digest for some people.

2. **Increased energy and improved mood:** Some people report feeling more energized and experiencing improved mood when they follow a gluten-free diet. However, there is limited scientific evidence to support these claims.

I believe eating correctly is like an investment for the future. We all want to live a long and healthy life, but sometimes we forget that our daily habits have a significant impact on our future health. Just as we invest in our financial future by managing our wealth, we should also invest in our health by managing our nutrition and lifestyle choices. Eating a healthy and balanced diet can help prevent many chronic diseases such as heart disease, diabetes, and obesity, and can improve our overall quality of life. Eating healthy now will help you to avoid chronic diseases, to maintain your energy levels, to build a stronger immune system, and to age gracefully.

Chapter 7
Summary

Overweight and obesity, as well as their related noncommunicable diseases, are largely preventable. Supportive environments and communities are fundamental in shaping children's choices.

Parents are advised by making the choice of healthier foods at home. And adopting regular physical activity is the easiest choice. At the adolescent age children/students can limit energy intake from total fats and sugars, increase consumption of fruit and vegetables, as well as legumes, whole grains and nuts; and engage in regular YOGA PRACTISES for 60 minutes a day.

The integrated Approach of Yoga Therapy which is incorporated in this book based on scientific research, having been practiced and adopted as a lifestyle will definitely help. This protocol if practiced in continuity will bring holistic changes based on five aspects of personality. This Module is designed on the basis of a literature review which is validated by 16 Yoga experts. It is effective in the management of weight, serum triglycerides and very low-density lipoprotein, hip circumference & serum cholesterol.
Yoga-based intervention is effective to reduce obesity in adolescents & children with respect to anthropometric, physical, psychological & cognitive assessments.

This book contains a research-based study that provides evidence to prove the efficacy of Yoga to manage increased subcutaneous adiposity in the trunk, hip and leg regions resulting in weight reduction in adolescent children and reducing abdominal circumference.

Yoga Practice helps in the reduction of Emotional overeating, enjoyment of food, desire to drink, food fussiness and satiety responsiveness. Regular practices of yoga protocol helps to improve good concentration, memory and attention. Yoga improves emotional well-being in children.

Yoga has been reported to have shown beneficial effects on different psychophysiological variables. Yoga is an ancient Indian science that helps to improve physical, mental, social and spiritual health. But many consider yoga as an alternative to exercise. There is a need to show that yoga is not merely an exercise system but it has many more health benefits. Our IAYT for adolescent obesity strictly follows this discipline. In our module, all Panchakoshas have been equally accessed which could be a guide for further studies.

Om Sarve Bhavantu Sukhinah,
Sarve Santu Niramaya,
Sarve Bhadrani Pashyantu,
Ma Kashchitt Dukha Bhag Bhavet.
Om Shantihi Shantihi Shantihi.
May All Be Happy and Prosperous,
May All Be Free from Illness,
May All Life Be Auspicious,
No One Becomes a Partaker of Sorrow.
Om Shanti, Shanti, Shanti.

Philosophy Behind Sarve Bhavantu Sukhinah Shloka. This "Om, Sarve Bhavantu Sukhinah" means "May everyone be happy" which means that everyone, every animal, every person and every atom, energy or whatever creature should be happy and free from suffering.

May all be free from diseases. May all see things auspicious. May none be subjected to misery. Om Shanti Shanti Shanti.

Read More

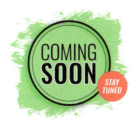
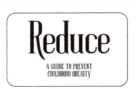

Reference

- Access, G., & Astrup, A. (2018). Fast-food habits, weight gain, and insulin resistance (the CARDIA study): 15-year prospective analysis. The Lancet, 365(9453), 4–5.

- Aggarwal, T., Bhatia, R. C., Singh, D., & Sobti, P. C. (2008). Prevalence of obesity and overweight in affluent adolescents from Ludhiana, Punjab. Indian Paediatrics, 45, 500–502.

- Ahima, R. S. (2011). Digging deeper into obesity Review series introduction. The Journal of Clinical Investigation, 121(6), 2076–2079. https://doi.org/10.1172/JCI58719

- Anwar, A., Anwar, F., Joiya, H. U., Ijaz, A., Rashid, H., Javaid, A., …Osmani, S. (2010). Prevalence of obesity among the school-going children of Lahore and associated factors. Journal of Ayub Medical College, 22(4), 27–32.

- Balasubramaniam, M., Telles, S., & Doraiswamy, P. M. (2013). Yoga on our minds : A systematic review of yoga for neuropsychiatric disorders. Frontiers in Psychiatry, Vol. 3. https://doi.org/10.3389/fpsyt.2012.00117

- Bashir, A. (2015). Effect of yogasanas practice on obesity of school going students in yavatmal city. International Research Journal of Physical Education and Sports Science, 2(2), 535–543.

- Benavides, S., & Caballero, J. (2009). Ashtanga yoga for children and adolescents for weight management and psychological well-being: An uncontrolled open pilot study. Complementary Therapies in Clinical Practice, 15, 110–114. https://doi. org/10.1016/j.ctcp.2008.12.004

- Bernstein, A. M., Bar, J., Ehrman, J. P., Golubic, M., & Roizen, M. F. (2014). Yoga in the Management of Overweight and Obesity. American Journal of Lifestyle Medicine, 8(1), 33–41. https://doi.org/10.1177/1559827613492097

- Carnell, S., & Wardle, J. (2007). Measuring behavioral susceptibility to obesity: Validation of the child eating behavior questionnaire. Appetite, 48(1), 104–113. https://doi.org/10.1016/J.APPET.2006.07.075

- Collins, C. E., Watson, J., & Burrows, T. (2010). Measuring dietary intake in children and adolescents in the context of overweight and obesity. International Journal of Obesity (2005), 34, 1103–1115. https://doi.org/10.1038/ijo.2009.241

- Dhananjai, S., Sadashiv, Tiwari, S., Dutt, K., & Kumar, R. (2013). Reducing psychological distress and obesity through Yoga practice. International Journal of

Yoga, 6, 66-70. https://doi. org/10.4103/09736131.105949

- Gaur, A., & Gupta, H. (2016). Incidence of Obesity among School Going Children of Urban and Rural Area of Moradabad - An Observational Study. Imperial Journal of Interdisciplinary Research, 2(10), 1259-1262.

- Goran, M. I. (2003). Obesity and Risk of Type 2 Diabetes and Cardiovascular Disease in Children and Adolescents. Journal of Clinical Endocrinology & Metabolism, 88(J. Clin. Endocrinol. Metab.), 1417-1427. https://doi.org/10.1210/jc.2002-021442

- H, T. S. Nn. (1994). Breathing through a particular nostril can alter metabolism and autonomic activities. No Title. Indian J Physiol Pharmacol., 38(2), 133-137.

- Hagen, I., & Nayar, U. S. (2014). Yoga for children and young people's mental health and well-being: Research review and reflections on the mental health potentials of yoga. Frontiers in Psychiatry, 5. https://doi.org/10.3389/fpsyt.2014.00035

- Haslam, D. W., & James, W. P. T. (2005a). Obesity. Lancet, 366, 1197-1209. https://doi.org/10.1016/S0140-6736(05)67483-1 Haslam, D. W., & James, W. P. T. (2005b). Obesity. The Lancet, 366(9492), 1197-1209. https://doi.org/10.1016/S0140-6736(05)67483-1

- Hu, F. B. (2008). Diet, Nutrition and Obesity. In Obesity Epidemiology (pp. 275-300).

- Inner engineering: book A yogi's guide to joy J Vasudev, Sadhguru- 2016 symdrik.com

- Jamesclear.com/atomic-habits/book

- Karnik, S., & Kanekar, A. (2012). Childhood obesity: A global public health crisis. International Journal of Preventive Medicine, 3, 1-7.

- Kelly, Cotter, E. W., & Mazzeo, S. E. (2012). Eating Disorder Examination Questionnaire (EDE-Q): Norms for Black women. Eating Behavio rs, 13, 429-432. rs, 13, 429-432. https://doi.org/10.1016/j.eatbeh.2012.09.001

- Khadilkar, V. V, Khadilkar, A. V, Cole, T. J., Chiplonkar, S. A., & Pandit, D. (2011). Overweight and obesity prevalence and body mass index trends in Indian children. International Journal of Paediatric Obesity, 6(2), e216-e224. https://doi.org/10.3 109/17477166.2010.541463

- Khalsa, S. B., & S., J.C.B.J.O.B.S.B.J.O.M.S. (2014). Yoga in public schools improves adolescent mood. Contemp School Psychological, 19(3), 184-192. Retrieved from 10.1007/s40688-014-0031-9

- Lee, H., Lee, I. S., & Choue, R. (2013). Obesity, Inflammation and Diet. Paediatric Gastroenterology, Hepatology & Nutrition, 16, 143-152. https://doi.org/10.5223/pghn.2013.16.3.143

- Lowe, M., & Fisher, E. B. J. (1983). Emotional reactivity, emotional eating, and obesity: A naturalistic study Title. Journal of Behavioural Medicine, 6(2), 135-149. Retrieved from https://doi.org/10.1007/ BF00845377

- Nagarathna, R., & Nagendra, H. . (2014). YOGA For OBESITY (First). Bangalore: Swami Vivekanad Vivekananda Yoga Prakashan.

- Nagendra, H. R., N. R. (1983). Application of integrated yoga. A Review. Yoga Review, 3, 173-194.

- Nagendra, H. R. (2006). Promotion of Positive Health. Bangalore: Swami Vivekananda Yoga Prakashana.

- Ogden, C., Carroll, M., Kit, B., & Flegal, K. (2014). Prevalence of childhood and adult obesity in the united states, 2011-2012. JAMA, 311(8), 806-814. Retrieved from http://dx.doi.org/10.1001/jama.2014.732

- Penny Gordon-Larsen. (2001). Obesity-Related Knowledge, Attitudes, and Behaviors in Obese and Non-obese Urban Philadelphia Female Adolescents - Gordon - Larsen - 2001 - Obesity Research - Wiley Online Library. Obesity & Research, 9(2), 112-118. Retrieved from https://onlinelibrary.wiley.com/doi/full/10.1038/oby.2001.1

- Prentice, A. M., & Jebb, S. A. (2001). Beyond body mass index. Obesity Reviews, 2, 141-147. https://doi.org/10.1046/ j.1467-789x.2001.00031.x

- Qi, L., & Cho, Y. A. (2008). Gene-environment interaction and obesity. Nutrition Reviews, Vol. 66, pp. 684-694. https://doi. org/10.1111/j.1753-4887.2008.00128.x

- Ranjani, H., Mehreen, T. S., Pradeepa, R., Anjana, R. M., Garg, R., Anand, K., & Mohan, V. (2016). Epidemiology of childhood overweight & obesity in India: A systematic review. Indian Journal of Medical Research, 143, 160-174. https://doi. org/10.4103/0971-5916.180203

- Rathi, S., Nagarathna, R., Nagendra, H. R., & Tekur, P. (2019). Feasibility study of integrated yoga module in overweight & obese adolescents. 12(4), 129-133. https://doi.org/10.15406/ijcam.2019.12.00462

- Rey-López, J. P., Vicente-Rodríguez, G., Biosca, M., & Moreno, L. A. (2008). Sedentary behavior and obesity development in children and adolescents. Nutrition, Metabolism, and Cardiovascular Diseases :, 18, 242-251. https://doi.org/10.1016/j. numecd.2007.07.008

- Rshikesan, P. B., Subramanya, P., & Nidhi, R. (2016). Yoga practice for reducing the male obesity and weight-related psychological difficulties A randomized controlled trial. Journal of Clinical and Diagnostic Research,10(11),OC22-OC28. https://doi.org/10.7860/JCDR/2016/22720.8940

- Rishikesan PB, S. P. (2016). Effect of integrated approach of yoga therapy on male obesity and psychological parameters – A randomized controlled trial. Journal of Clinical and Diagnostic Research, 10(10), KC01-KC06. https://doi.org/10.7860/

- S, D. (2009). Complications of obesity in children and adolescents. International Journal of Obesity, 33(1), S60–S65. https:// doi.org/10.1038/ijo.2009.20

- Seo, D. Y., Lee, S., Figueroa, A., Kim, H. K., Baek, Y. H., Kwak, Y. S., ... Han, J. (2012). Yoga training improves metabolic parameters in obese boys. Korean Journal of Physiology and Pharmacology, 16(3), 175–180. https://doi.org/10.4196/ kjpp.2012.16.3.175

- Seth, A., & Sharma, R. (2013). Childhood obesity. Indian Journal of Paediatrics, pp. 309–317. Retrieved from https:doi.10.1007/s 12098-012-0935-5

- Telles S, Nagarathna R, N. H. R. (2008). Physiological Measures of Right Nostril Breathing. The Journal of Alternative and Complementary Medicine, 2(4). Retrieved from https://doi.org/10.1089/acm.1996.2.479

- Telles, S., Gaur, V., & Balkrishna, A. (2009). Effect of a yoga practice session and a yoga theory session on state anxiety. Perceptual and Motor Skills, Vol. 109, pp. 924–930.Retrieved from https://www.ncbi.nlm.nih.gov/pubmed/20178291

- Telles, S., Nagarathna, R., & Nagendra, H. R. (1994). Breathing through a particular nostril can alter metabolism and autonomic activities. Indian Journal of Physiology and Pharmacology, 38, 133–137.

- Telles, S., Narendran, S., Raghuraj, P., Nagarathna, R., & Nagendra, H. R. (1997). Comparison of changes in autonomic and respiratory parameters of girls after yoga and games at a community home. Perceptual and Motor Skills, 84(1), 251–257. https://doi.org/10.2466pms.1997.84.1.251

- Telles, S., Naveen, V. K., Balkrishna, A., & Kumar, S. (2010). Short-term health impact of a yoga and diet change program on obesity. Medical Science Monitor: International Medical Journal of Experimental and Clinical Research, 16(1), CR3540.

- Telles, S., Naveen, V., Science, A. B.-M., & 2009, U. (2009). Short-term health impact of a yoga and diet change program on obesity. Medscimonit.Com, 15(12). Retrieved from https://www.medscimonit.com/abstract/index/idArt/878317/new/1/ act/3

- Telles, S., Singh, N., Bhardwaj, A. K., Kumar, A., & Balkrishna, A. (2013). Effect of yoga or physical exercise on physical, cognitive and emotional measures in children: a randomized controlled trial. Child and Adolescent Psychiatry and Mental Health, 7(1), 37. Retrieved from http://www.pubmedcentral.nih.gov/articlerender.fcgi?artid=3826528&tool=pmcentrez&rendertype=abstract

- Telles, S., Singh, N., Kumar, A. B., Kumar, A., & Balkrishna, A. (2013). Effect of yoga or physical exercise on physical, cognitive and emotional measures in children: a randomized controlled trial. Child and Adolescent Psychiatry and Mental

- Health, 7, 37. https://doi.org/10.1186/1753-2000-7-37

- Thakur, K. (2013). Effects of Surya Namaskara on Selected Psychological Parameters of School Boys. International Journal of Health Sciences and Research (IJHSR), 3, 65–69.

- Thivel, D., Tremblay, M. S., & Chaput, J.-P. (2013). Modern Sedentary Behaviors Favour Energy Consumption in Children and Adolescents. Current Obesity Reports, 2(1), 50–57. https://doi.org/10.1007/s13679-012-0032-9

- Vallath Nandini. (2010). Perspectives on Yoga Inputs in the Management of Chronic PainNo Title. Indian J Palliat Care., 16(1), 1–7.

- Van Der Kruk, J. J., Kortekaas, F., Lucas, C., & Jager-Wittenaar, H. (2013). Obesity: A systematic review on parental involvement in long-term European childhood weight control interventions with a nutritional focus. Obesity Reviews, 14,

- 745–760. https://doi.org/10.1111/obr.12046

- Webber, L., Hill, C., Saxton, J., Van Jaarsveld, C. H. M., & Wardle, J. (2009). PAEDIATRIC HIGHLIGHT Eating behavior and weight in children. International Journal of Obesity, 33(1), 21–28. https://doi.org/10.1038/ijo.2008.219

- WHO. (2000). Obesity: preventing and managing the global epidemic. Report of a WHO consultation. World Health Organization Technical Report Series, 894, i–xii, 1–253. Retrieved from http://www.ncbi.nlm.nih.gov/pubmed/11234459 WHO.

Co-Author's Bio

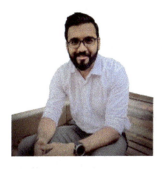

Introducing " Reduce - A Guide to Prevent Childhood Obesity" by Dr. Sunanda Rathi & Mr. Aashish S Rathi In a world that often rushes us through the chaos of daily life, where stress and unhealthy habits seem to lurk around every corner, the quest for a balanced and healthy lifestyle becomes a paramount necessity.

In the pages of "Reduce - A Guide to Prevent Childhood Obesity" we are introduced to Mr. Aashish S Rathi, a remarkable individual whose life story is a testament to the power of embracing a holistic approach to health and well-being.

Aashish is an entrepreneur, an educational counselor, a sports enthusiast, a public speaker, and, above all, a firm believer in the profound benefits of a healthy lifestyle. His journey through life has been shaped by a commitment to wellness that goes beyond mere physical fitness. It is a philosophy that permeates every aspect of his existence, from his career choices to his personal practices.

Aashish's professional journey is as inspiring as his dedication to health. Having served as an Assistant Manager in the IT sector with KEC International Limited, he transitioned to become the operational head at an Animation training academy. But what truly sets him apart is his vision to create countless job opportunities in the exciting realms of animation, VFX, gaming, and comic design. His passion for these industries goes hand-in-hand with his commitment to empowering the youth, motivating them with a positive and solution-oriented approach.

Educated in computer science at Pune University, Aashish went on to earn a MBA in IT from I2IT, Pune, and a diploma in business finance. He is an active member of BNI, the world's largest networking organization, and Maheshwari Vidya Pracharak Mandal (MVPM), a trust dedicated to helping students excel in education and sports through various initiatives. Additionally, he is affiliated with the Indian Yoga Association (IYA), further demonstrating his holistic approach to well-being.

Aashish's dedication to health and fitness is undeniable, backed by his certification in sports nutrition and exercise science from Get Set Go Fitness. He's not just a proponent of healthy living; he's a practitioner who understands the profound impact of nutrition and physical activity on one's overall vitality.

Beyond the boardrooms and fitness studios, Aashish S Rathi is a true sports enthusiast. He's a national-level roller skater, an active cricket player at PYC, and has represented his alma mater, Fergusson College, in inter-college football matches. His talents extend to baseball and softball, where he's competed at the state level.

In the realm of spiritual guidance, Aashish follows the teachings of Sadhguru and Mahatrias, finding solace and wisdom in their practices.

Moreover, his journey as a father to a toddler has brought an added layer of meaning to his pursuit of a healthy lifestyle. Over the past four years, he has not only preached but lived by the principle that "you are what you eat," mindfully incorporating wellness into his family's daily life.

"Reduce" is more than just a book; it's an invitation to embark on a transformative path towards a healthier, more fulfilling life. Aashish S Rathi's story serves as a beacon of inspiration, offering practical insights and invaluable wisdom for those who seek to enhance their physical, mental, and emotional well-being. Whether you're an aspiring entrepreneur, a sports enthusiast, a parent, or simply someone eager to embrace a healthier lifestyle, this book is your guide to holistic wellness and a testament to the transformative power of choice.

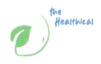

Author's Bio

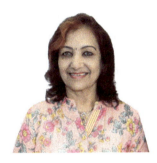

Dr. Sunanda Rathi is a distinguished academician and yog researcher with a diverse educational background. She holds a Ph.D. in Communication & Business Management, a Bachelor of Law, and a Master of Commerce, from Pune University.

In the world of wellness, education, and holistic healing, Dr. Rathi stands as a beacon of knowledge and compassion. With a rich tapestry of academic accomplishments and a deep-rooted commitment to social well-being, her journey has been nothing short of inspiring. As an esteemed academician and a distinguished yog researcher, Dr. Rathi has dedicated her life to understanding and harnessing the power of yog, communication, and business management to benefit individuals and communities alike.

Her thirst for understanding the intricate connection between mind, body, and soul led her to pursue another Ph.D. in Yog from S-Vyasa, Bangalore. Her research delved into the "Effect of Integrated Approach of Yoga Therapy on Adolescent Obesity." This profound exploration illuminated the potential of yoga as a holistic approach to combating one of the pressing health concerns of our time. Dr. Rathi's groundbreaking work in developing a protocol for obesity has garnered attention from schools in Maharashtra. The adoption of her protocol has yielded fantastic results, effectively reduced fat and enhancing mental and physical well-being among students. This initiative is a testament to her dedication to promoting healthier lifestyles among the youth.

She has also completed different courses from esteemed institutes to deepen her insights.

Her quest for knowledge has not only been personal but also altruistic. In 2016, she founded the Chiranjiv Foundation: Yog Education & Research a platform that embodies her vision to disseminate the wisdom of yog for the betterment of the community. Driven by an experienced and dedicated team, this foundation has become a bastion of excellence in creating pool of certified Yog Instructor.

One of the most commendable aspects of Dr. Rathi's work is her unwavering commitment to the well-being of children with special needs. By providing specialized trainers and establishing a consistent routine, she empowers these children to improve their physical, mental, and emotional health, offering them a path to greater well-being and integration into society.

Dr. Rathi's contributions extend far and wide, touching various facets of society. Her numerous awards and honours, including the Rajeev Gandhi Excellence Award and Yuwa Bharati Award, bear testament to her dedication and hard work in the field of social service.

Alongside her contributions to the field of yoga, Dr. Rathi has established several professional ventures. She founded Arena Animation Tilak Road in 1997, an institute specializing in multimedia and animation training which offers premium training in graphics, website design, digital marketing, 2D and 3D animation, visual effects, and live-action movies having job opportunities across various industries.

In addition to her work in education, Dr. Rathi's impact on healthcare and wellness is significant. Her role as a Senior Research Fellow for the Ministry of AYUSH's Diabetes Project in Maharashtra and Goa underscores her dedication to healthcare advancements. Her membership in the Scientific Advisory Research Committee of SPPU reflects her commitment to academic excellence and scientific research.

Furthermore, her role as a Content Developer for Ramkumar Rathi Patanjali Yoga Chair, online courses showcase her dedication to knowledge dissemination in the digital age.

Dr. Sunanda Rathi's multifaceted roles and contributions in healthcare, education, and research have left a lasting impact on the communities she serves. Dr. Rathi is not just an author but a catalyst for transformation.

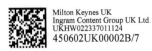
Milton Keynes UK
Ingram Content Group UK Ltd.
UKHW022337011124
450602UK00002B/7